Surviving and Thriving

Confronting Systemic Omissions and Impacts in Educational Policy

Shaheen Shariff
General Editor

Vol. 3

The Confronting Systemic Omissions and
Impacts in Educational Policy series is
part of the Peter Lang Education list.

Every volume is peer reviewed and meets the
highest quality standards for content and production.

PETER LANG

New York · Berlin · Bruxelles · Chennai · Lausanne · Oxford

Surviving and Thriving

Promoting Health and Well-being During and After COVID-19

Shaheen Shariff, Christopher Dietzel,
Safia Amiry, Safeera Jaffer

PETER LANG

New York · Berlin · Bruxelles · Chennai · Lausanne · Oxford

Library of Congress Cataloging-in-Publication Data
Print LCCN: 2025015786

Bibliographic information published by the Deutsche Nationalbibliothek.
The German National Library lists this publication in the German
National Bibliography; detailed bibliographic data is available
on the Internet at http://dnb.d-nb.de.

This work was supported by iMPACTS: Collaborations to Address Sexual Violence
on Campus; Social Sciences and Humanities Research Council (SSHRC) of Canada
Partnership Grant Number: 895-2016-1026, Project Director, Shaheen Shariff, Ph.D.,
James McGill Professor, McGill University.

Artwork by Shaheen Shariff, Cover Design by Alyssa Jetha

ISSN 2834-6939
ISBN 978-3-0343-5243-7 (print)
ISBN 978-3-0343-5422-6 (ePDF)
ISBN 978-3-0343-5423-3 (ePub)
DOI 10.3726/b22899

This publication has been peer reviewed.

Dedication from Shaheen Shariff, Ph.D.

For my incredible team of graduate and post-graduate
Research Associates and Research Assistants. I know that
each of you will succeed in your careers because of your work ethic,
insight, and dedication.

Dedication from Christopher Dietzel, Ph.D.

To the many individuals and communities who have felt the impacts
of the COVID-19 pandemic exacerbated by systems of inequity.

Dedication from Safia Amiry

To my father, whose unwavering love and enduring confidence in me
have shaped the person I am today.

Dedication from Safeera Jaffer

To all the people who experience the ongoing COVID-19 pandemic
as intricately tied to other systems of oppression. While these forces
are connected, so too is liberation.

TABLE OF CONTENTS

PREFACE BY THE EDITORS

In the years since the emergence of COVID-19, the world has experienced unprecedented changes. Concerns about viral transmission during the pandemic forced people to work from home and students to attend virtual classes. Government-imposed lockdowns often prohibited people from meeting in person, or placed restrictions on how people could gather. During that unprecedented global crisis, societal systems were pushed to their limits and individuals confronted novel risks to their health—not only because of this new virus and its long-term health consequences, but also because of the impacts that pandemic-related conditions had on people's well-being, social interactions, and quality of life.

As the world has shifted from the urgent threats related to the COVID-19 pandemic, it is crucial to recognize that the novel coronavirus, along with pandemic-related impacts, have not disappeared. The pandemic's effects continue to influence people's everyday lives, especially those who are part of marginalized communities.

Health justice is an important concept to consider due to the multiple, complex, and interlocking inequities and inequalities that were exposed—and exacerbated—because of the COVID-19 pandemic. Defined as both a theoretical framework and movement to eliminate health inequities, health justice is important because it emphasizes ethics of care surrounding the relationships between health, public health, and the root causes of health inequity (Wiley et al., 2022). Social justice is a core aspect of health justice (Wiley et al., 2022), and with this more critical and equity-focused lens, we can see that the lingering health impacts of the COVID-19 pandemic are distinctly tied to other forces of power and oppression. This is not surprising, given that numerous studies have revealed the disproportionate impact of the pandemic on various, and often historically marginalized, populations (Borras, 2021). Factors such as age, race, gender, sexual orientation, dis/ability, and socio-economic background, among others, have been shown to alter how different populations experienced the pandemic, including threats to their physical, mental, and social health, and have shed light on lasting health impacts post-pandemic (Bowleg, 2020; Lei & Guo, 2022; Lund et al., 2020). Of course, this should not be surprising since, as noted above, the pandemic revealed and amplified the health inequities that are embedded throughout society. A health justice framework, therefore, pushes us to scrutinize what happened during the pandemic and critically consider empirical, equitable solutions that can be applied to mitigate and prevent future health injustices, whether during a time of crisis or in general.

It is with such a vision that we approached this edited collection. We sought to analyze, through an intersectional and health justice-oriented framework, the health inequities and inequalities that were exposed and exacerbated during the COVID-19 pandemic and offer evidence-based recommendations that could be applied to various sectors of society—not just within the fields of healthcare. As such, this edited collection brings together research related to the health and well-being of various populations, including people who experience homelessness, children and youth, young perfectionists, and students enrolled in health professions education. Examining the roles of homelessness, arts-based participatory research, perfectionism, maltreatment disclosures, and educational programming, the authors in this edited collection explore various health-related issues that children, youth, and adults faced during the pandemic.

As noted above, our goal with this edited collection is not simply to examine these health inequities. Instead, we intend to mitigate harmful health-related consequences by offering specific, meaningful recommendations relevant to health promotion, policy, and education, among other areas of society, and by sharing important reflections for future actions. Thus, this edited collection provides key lessons and relevant insights into health impacts of the COVID-19 pandemic and encourages the reader to apply this knowledge to address ongoing and emerging challenges.

Chapter 1—A Disaster Within a Disaster: Homelessness During the COVID-19 Pandemic

In the book's first chapter written by Jeff Karabanow, Jean Hughes, Haorui Wu, and Catherine Leviten-Reid, the authors analyze the effects of the pandemic on two major groups in Nova Scotia, Canada: people experiencing homelessness and stakeholders such as service workers and government officials who work in the area of homelessness. While homelessness already included disastrous, long-term consequences, the public health emergency of the COVID-19 pandemic magnified and heightened these challenges on individual, community, and policy levels. Through this qualitative case study, the authors reveal how the COVID-19 pandemic exacerbated physical and mental struggles for people experiencing homelessness. This group was also often overlooked by public health and safety measures. Service stakeholders also faced several challenges in their work, but the authors share how bringing together workers in the health and housing sectors deepened partnerships and collaboration. In the future, creative and quick mobilization of collaborative efforts along with affordable, sustainable, and supportive housing will be critical to develop solutions and support people experiencing homelessness.

Chapter 2—A Reflexive Account of Facilitating an Online Study of the Pandemic Experiences of Canadian Youth Using Cellphilms

Through an analysis of their online research with Canadian youth during the COVID-19 pandemic, Grace Skahan, S. M. Hani Sadati, Shannon Roy, and Claudia Mitchell describe their personal reflections and findings from their qualitative, arts-based participatory framework and *cellphilming methodology* (cellphone + film). Through facilitating online workshops, the authors learned from youth how the pandemic affected them and how they dealt with various challenges. One of the major findings included the prevalence of stress and mental health struggles such as depression, insomnia, and anxiety for youth during the pandemic. In addition to these direct findings from youth, this study provided important insights into the experience of conducting research online during a pandemic situation.

Chapter 3—"They're Kind of Losing It": Young Perfectionists' Mental Health Experiences During the First COVID-19 Lockdown

Chapter 3 by Dawn Zinga, Danielle S. Molnar, Melissa Blackburn, and Natalie Tacuri addresses how the pandemic affected the mental health of self-identified perfectionists in Ontario, Canada. The study reveals how perfectionist youth may experience more challenges during the pandemic compared to their non perfectionistic peers. The study provides an in-depth understanding of the unique challenges experienced by young perfectionists and the strategies that helped them to cope with mental health concerns. The authors also emphasize the fact that perfectionistic youth were already grappling with mental health challenges before the pandemic and will likely still have difficulties afterwards. This chapter highlights the urgent need for targeted strategies and rigorous attention to help perfectionistic youth effectively navigate mental health challenges.

Chapter 4—Disclosures of Child Maltreatment Through Computer-Mediated Communication: A Call to Action

This chapter underscores the role of computer-mediated communication (CMC) in facilitating disclosure of child maltreatment and abuse. It draws attention to how stay-at-home policies during the COVID-19 pandemic contributed significantly to higher rates of abuse, loneliness, and mental health issues that Canadian children experienced. As a result, there is a greater dependence on CMC tools for social interaction. Given the recent rise in reports of child maltreatment, mental health problems, and increased usage of CMC, it is likely that a greater number of children are reporting abuse experiences through CMC. As a result, the authors Olivia Leslie Holden, Annie Yun An Shiau, Shayla Chilliak, Victoria Talwar, and Shanna DeWit Williams call for further research in this area, especially after the height of the pandemic, to fully understand CMC's function as a tool for reporting abuse and maltreatment.

Chapter 5—Recommendations to Mitigate Future Pandemic Impacts on Health Professions Education: Lessons Learned During the COVID-19 Pandemic

The fifth and final chapter of this edited collection authored by Kelly Lackie, Neda Alizadeh, Mark Embrett, Simon Field, Jennifer Lane, Marion Brown, Diane MacKenzie, Bright Huo, Kathleen MacMillan, and Ruth Martin-Misener explores the difficulties that health education, specifically skill-based learning programs, faced in Nova Scotia during the COVID-19 pandemic. The transition of these programs to online modalities not only affected educational delivery, but it also raised concerns regarding the programs' efficacy in developing students' professional abilities and sufficiently preparing them for safe practice in their respective disciplines. The study's findings highlight a wide range of strategies used by different institutions to navigate the challenge presented by the pandemic. Institutions showed flexibility to meet changing student needs while abiding by health guidelines. Despite the adjustments made by different programs, students voiced doubts about their potential for success in the workplace. Students' confidence in their ability to proficiently develop skills declined due to the shift in the practical learning opportunities. However, the study also highlighted the importance of extracurricular healthcare activities, which proved to be useful for some students to maintain interest and improve their skills in their respective professions. To further improve the resilience of the health education system, this final chapter offers a thorough set of recommendations for education providers and other stakeholders as a road map to strengthen the system against comparable obstacles in the future, ensuring sustained quality in training healthcare workers in the constantly changing field of healthcare delivery.

Bibliography

Borras, A. M. (2021). Toward an intersectional approach to health justice. *International Journal of Health Services, 51*(2), 206–225.

Bowleg, L. (2020). We're not all in this together: On COVID-19, intersectionality, and structural inequality. *American Journal of Public Health, 110*(7), 917.

Lei, L., & Guo, S. (2022). Beyond multiculturalism: Revisioning a model of pandemic anti-racism education in post-Covid-19 Canada. *International Journal of Anthropology and Ethnology, 6*(1), 1–22.

Lund, E. M., Forber-Pratt, A. J., Wilson, C., & Mona, L. R. (2020). The COVID-19 pandemic, stress, and trauma in the disability community: A call to action. *Rehabilitation Psychology, 65*(4), 313–322.

Wiley, L. F., Yearby, R., Clark, B. R., & Mohapatra, S. (2022). Introduction: What is health justice? *The Journal of Law, Medicine & Ethics: A Journal of the American Society of Law, Medicine & Ethics, 50*(4), 636–640.

A DISASTER WITHIN A DISASTER: HOMELESSNESS DURING THE COVID-19 PANDEMIC

Jeff Karabanow, Jean Hughes,
Haorui Wu, and Catherine Leviten-Reid

Introduction

This chapter discusses the COVID-19-driven impacts on two interrelated groups within the homelessness sector in the two largest municipalities in Nova Scotia (NS)—Halifax Regional Municipality (HRM) and Cape Breton Regional Municipality (CBRM): 1) persons experiencing homelessness (PEHs) who are connected to community organizations that partnered with the research team and 2) stakeholders (service providers and governmental officials) who were working in the area of homelessness. A background on homelessness will first be provided, along with the identification of stakeholders in NS who are involved with supporting those experiencing homelessness. Attention will then focus on the impact of the COVID-19 pandemic on these two groups, highlighting the unique challenges experienced by both. The research involved a qualitative study employing a case study approach using a constant comparative method. The chapter will close with a discussion on lessons learned during the COVID-19 pandemic and recommendations to ensure a more cohesive response in the event of future emergencies.

Background

Homelessness is a situation in which an individual, family, or community does not have stable or appropriate housing (Karabanow et al., 2023). There are broad categories included under the umbrella term of "homeless," involving unsheltered (e.g., living in public places or a car), emergency sheltered (e.g., stop-gap shelters designed for short-term stays), provisionally accommodated (e.g., access to short-term, non-permanent accommodation without the prospect of permanent housing), and risk of homelessness (e.g., people who are housed but faced with the possibility of losing this accommodation) (Gaetz et al., 2012). Within Canada, approximately 3% of the population has experienced homelessness (Uppal, 2022). This number is increasing year by year across the country.

An important contextual consideration is that homelessness itself is a disastrous status, which is not a short-term, unanticipated extreme event, but a structural, long-term, and neglected phenomenon associated with a full spectrum of societal dimensions (e.g., economic, social, health, cultural, and political) (Wu et al., 2022). The experience of homelessness is dehumanizing, unforgiving, dire and yields devastating consequences (Corburn et al., 2020; Perri et al., 2020). The vast majority of PEHs encounter daily struggles, trauma, and consistent stress and fear when seeking some form of survival, shelter, food, connection, income, and/or security (Karabanow et al., 2018). The diversity and complexity of homelessness create a scenario in which unexpected disruptions or strain on society and/or resources can have a disastrous effect on an already strained healthcare and social service system. One such event was the COVID-19 pandemic.

The global public health emergency of the COVID-19 pandemic increased different societal pressure on PEHs (Karabanow et al., 2022). The public health mitigation strategies, such as social distancing and lockdown, prevented PEHs from accessing essential services, such as hygiene facilities (e.g., washrooms and showers) and food banks (Doll et al., 2022). At the community level, PEH-specific community-based service agencies such as homeless shelters and substance use support did not have the emergency response capacity to swiftly adjust their service delivery, leaving most PEHs unserved at the immediate outset of the pandemic (Gin et al., 2022). Although these grassroots struggles stimulate human rights advocacy for PEHs and further inform related service programs and policies, the voices of PEH tend to be ignored in decision and policy-making processes, especially those associated with the long-term PEH-specific societal issues, such as affordable housing, poverty reduction, and accessible healthcare and social services (Karabanow et al., 2023). These three issues regarding homelessness suggest threefold interventions to support PEHs at the individual (micro), community/organization (mezzo), and program/policy (macro) levels; namely, addressing their unique requirements through individual and/or organizational support and developing PEH-driven program and policies (Zufferey & Parkes, 2019). These three-level interventions are the foundation of social work efforts, collaborating with diverse stakeholders to reduce PEH's vulnerabilities and enhance their health and well-being, ultimately contributing to just societies (Manthorpe et al., 2015).

Stakeholders who play a role in supporting PEHs and working toward housing security are instrumental in trying to rectify the homelessness disaster. Within NS, HRM and CBRM were of interest to study because their disparate geographical locations and resources afforded the opportunity to understand what challenges and opportunities are unique to or shared by these communities. At the beginning of the COVID crisis, HRM and CBRM brought together their own service providers (such as shelters, drop-in services, health clinics, and street outreach) alongside municipal personnel, provincial government employees, public health officials, and federal funders with the goal of better understanding how these organizations supported the homeless population during the COVID-19 pandemic. These groups became known as the COVID-19 Tables. One important difference is that HRM involved more decision makers and is seen as more central to government resources because Halifax is the capital city. CBRM is a 5-hour drive away from the capital and reflects more rural and remote communities.

The following sections are a reflection and analysis of a study that was conducted by Karabanow et al. (2023) (see also Doll et al., 2022) during the COVID-19 pandemic to critically understand the lived experience of the homeless population in HRM and CBRM in response to the COVID-19 pandemic. Furthermore, the response of key stakeholders in supporting the homeless population of these regions is discussed in terms of challenges that were encountered and considerations that might facilitate a more coordinated and compassionate response to supporting people experiencing homelessness during a global and even local crisis. This chapter, in essence, speaks to lessons learned from the COVID-19 pandemic regarding preventive actions that can hopefully be replicated in other disasters and within other communities.

Methods

This chapter employs a case study approach to explore stakeholders within the homelessness sector in two study settings of HRM and CBRM during the first wave of COVID-19 in NS (March-May 2020). The Social Sciences and Humanities Research Ethics Board at Dalhousie University approved this research, as did the Research Ethics Board at Cape Breton University.

Study Settings

HRM, including two cities of Halifax and Dartmouth with surrounding suburban communities, had a total population of 448,544 in 2021 (Government of Canada, 2022). CBRM featured a population of 93,694, and includes one urban center (Sydney) and surrounding suburban and rural communities (Government of Canada, 2022). Although HRM and CBRM's geographical locations are distinct, they both feature collaborative relationships among stakeholders (i.e., PEHs and service stakeholders).

Research Participants

Two interrelated groups within the homelessness sector were invited to participate in this research. First, PEHs who were connected to community organizations that partnered with the research team were invited. Secondly, service stakeholders who were working in the area of housing and homelessness—such as shelter providers, health clinic workers, outreach personnel, housing advocates, public health workers, policy makers, and government representatives—were also invited to participate. In total, 28 PEHs and 24 service stakeholders were recruited. The perspectives from both groups built a two-way approach to deeply understand PEHs' challenges and the experiences of service stakeholders.

Data Collection

Semi-structured, individual, in-depth interviews were employed to obtain data, representing a snapshot of the homelessness sector and a snapshot of the pandemic. Open-ended interview questions were asked to help the participants to reflect on their experiences from the time the pandemic was declared to the time they sat down to be interviewed. The interviews with most service stakeholders were conducted by phone or video conferencing, while interviews with those experiencing homelessness were conducted in person at two community-based sites. Each interview, ranging from 30 minutes to one hour, was audio recorded.

Data Analysis

The verbatim transcription was obtained from each interview and analyzed by the research team using an approach called "the constant comparative method." This qualitative data analysis approach aims to identify common themes in the data by first assigning codes to interview transcriptions and then grouping these codes into larger sub-themes. These sub-themes are grouped into major themes in an iterative process (Strauss & Corbin, 1990). To strengthen the validity of the findings, the team members independently analyzed each transcription through developing codes and sub-themes. They collaboratively developed themes through group discussion. Through this chapter, the participants' quotations were provided to support different sub-themes and themes. Many of the themes that surfaced from our data are similar to research findings on homelessness and disasters in other locations such as the United States and Australia (Osborn et al., 2019; Pixley et al., 2022).

Results

In reviewing transcripts, we found two main overarching narratives. The vast majority of participants, both PEHs and service stakeholders, expressed overwhelming feelings of frustration, tiredness, uncertainty, and hurt. Yet, at the same time, these groups also spoke about survival, passion, and strength. As one PEH noted to our team: "I appreciate the time and consideration that you take … You actually take the time to give a shit about us." Our participants need to be heard, and their voices can help prepare for future emergency operations. As one service stakeholder noted, "I think it's very important that we sketch something around a road map." What follows are the core themes that make up the most relevant narratives for a group of individuals experiencing homelessness throughout the pandemic and service providers tasked with developing, supporting, innovating, and funding a strategic disaster response.

The Effect of the COVID-19 Pandemic on PEHs

The Impact of COVID-19 Public Health Measures

The COVID-19 pandemic for the most part amplified the suffering of being homeless. The nature of this pandemic increased levels of stress, anxiety, fear, and uncertainty within the population. As one PEH noted, "It affected me really bad over the last year, like mentally wise, like physically, physically and mentally, it did … It's real hard over the last year." There was also an atmosphere of uncertainty and one PEH indicated that: "Like I was just scared always." The struggle of daily life for PEHs was magnified by the collective uncertainty around the COVID-19 pandemic, which, accordingly, intensified the already difficult experience of those without housing.

While being homeless itself can be extremely vulnerable, unsafe, harrowing and exhausting, the COVID-19 pandemic increased the feeling of marginalization, isolation, loneliness, stigma, lack of control, and physical, emotional, psychological, and spiritual strain. Many PEHs who were interviewed during the COVID-19 pandemic found it to be "a dire, hopeless situation" and commented on "depression, stress, lack of appetite. Stress and stuff from all this shit." One participant summed up the common feeling: "Feels like you have no support." Many spoke of feeling "isolated," "forgotten," and "helpless," with one participant stating that "the isolation was such a big piece for everybody."

Most participants experiencing homelessness spoke about being deeply "exposed" and "left behind." Living rough entails living out one's private world in public spaces (Karabanow, 2006). However, when public spaces are closed down, homelessness takes on a more disastrous tone from a lack of public facilities, lack of water and bathroom (usually obtained by dropping into a nearby restaurant/café or library), lack of service provider support (many organizations closing down or moving to a virtual platform of care), lack of transportation (buses shut down for some time), and lack of congregate, common space for daily connection (a good example is the closure of libraries and parks) (Doll et al., 2022; Karabanow et al., 2022). This has a ruthless impact on an already tired and scared population.

Public Health Measures and Access to Information

The main public health rallying calls in NS (and in retrospect throughout the world) involved "stay home," "wash your hands," "wear a mask," and "socially distance" (Province of NS, 2020; Wu & Karabanow, 2020). As noted by a service stakeholder: "those directives were so out of touch with a population that had no home." For those living rough (e.g., in parks, on the street, and/or in abandoned buildings) and at formal and informal shelters, these ordinances were simply unattainable. As noted by a PEH: "Where was I going to sleep that night, where was I going to eat, where was I going to relax? Pretty much where was I going to rest my head at night?" PEHs did not have homes to stay in; they did not have easy access to water, washrooms, or sinks; most often they could not acquire masks; and it was almost impossible to have any distance in shelters (Doll et al., 2022). A PEH shared that "[COVID] hit us even harder, because we were like, being homeless you're outside, you are around other people constantly, constantly around other people." The vast majority of PEHs spoke about the added difficulties involved in finding food, safe living arrangements, any form of employment, a safe supply of protective masks, and being updated on COVID-19 in the midst of a powerful pandemic that stifled movement and community. As such, we find a population in more struggle for connection and support.

Many PEHs also felt uninformed about the pandemic due to a severe lack of communication and knowledge transfer. For many, access to social media, news outlets, the internet, and friends and family was severely hampered by the COVID-19 pandemic. A PEH described the feeling of being disconnected as follows:

> Everyone should have at least a phone or access to a communication device … that should be a free service … for every reason … emergency or not … and if you are that low and your only possession is a telephone, well most of the time you are living in an emergency in a way right? … And that's why it is so important for anybody that's homeless to be able to communicate.

This feeling of disconnection within the homeless community was pervasive before the COVID-19 pandemic, but when previously available sources of connection were disrupted by public health measures, the feeling of isolation was magnified. Clearly, as has also been found in other countries (Ralli et al., 2021), PEHs in NS were overlooked by safety and health monitoring actions enacted during the COVID-19 pandemic, primarily staying inside one's residence, wearing masks, and being able to socially isolate. These public health measures placed them at high risk of being left behind.

A Pandemic Response: The Story of Service Stakeholders

Initial Response to the COVID-19 Pandemic

PEHs were not the only ones who articulated strong emotions when the pandemic hit. From the interviews we conducted with service stakeholders from the COVID-Tables, the majority of service stakeholders spoke about the feelings of "fear," "stress," "uncertainty," and "confusion" that made up the early days of the pandemic. A service stakeholder indicated that "It was very, very, scary," "extremely challenging," and many experienced "a heightened sense of anxiety and concern." Service stakeholders expressed a sense of "chaos," "shock," and at first "not knowing what to do." Several participants noted that these were extremely "challenging times" with public health dictates that "changed consistently," especially in terms of how to keep staff and clients safe (e.g., protocol concerning group congregation and mask wearing). One service stakeholder was clear to say that the early days of the COVID-19 pandemic were best characterized as "a shit show." Reflecting on the first wave of the pandemic, all service stakeholders around the Tables noted how "lucky" it was that there was very little spread of the virus within the homeless community in NS—a testament to not only luck but some very significant actions taken by members of these Tables, as will be described below. One service stakeholder reflected that "we were also extremely lucky and well mobilized that the spread [of COVID] didn't happen in the homeless community." While of course

PEH did contract COVID-19, this excerpt speaks to infections not rapidly being transmitted among those experiencing homelessness as they did, for example, in some long-term care facilities where people are older and live close to one another.

Service stakeholders unanimously agreed that the pandemic shed light on the existing and growing crises of homelessness, lack of affordable housing, poverty, food insecurity, dearth of employment/income, and social connection. A service stakeholder noted that "there's been a bit more of a kind of increased awareness to the struggles this population [PEHs] is facing ... a broader acknowledgment of how this population is vulnerable and marginalized." As will be discussed later, through this increased visibility of PEHs via the closure of facilities they typically accessed, as well as greater media attention on homelessness, the necessity of stable housing as a human right has now permeated into the daily conversations of the general public. In this context, there is a possibility to enact change, as collective action can be taken by communities who feel they can relate in a more humanistic manner to PEHs.

Involvement of Public Health

According to several service stakeholder participants, prior to the COVID-19 pandemic, public health had very little to do with the homeless sector and as one service stakeholder noted, "homeless populations tended to be ignored by public health." Yet, it was not uncommon for topics around the social determinants of health to surface in Service Table discussions. Since the COVID-19 pandemic was defined as a health issue, public health was brought to these discussions, which was a first-time occurrence for many of those working in this arena. Public health employees and service stakeholders later acknowledged the vast learning curve experienced as both sectors (housing and health) shared their expertise. For example, shelter workers often noted that their clients were picking up cigarette butts, which was extremely risky during the pandemic. Public health employees offered nicotine replacement supplies in response, which shelter workers knew would not have buy-in from their clients. In the end, funds were found to purchase cigarettes as a harm reduction solution. Both sectors felt that there was deep learning here in terms of taking a collaborative approach to care, as summarized by a service stakeholder that "oh yeah, like so collaboration and relationships [emerged] ... you know sharing knowledge of what each of us does."

The involvement of public health at the Tables was seen as a significant addition because their presence provided a health lens to the discussions. As provincial health protocols developed and changed, public health members were available to provide the groups with support and guidance. For example, public health officials visited shelters to explore ways in which collective spaces could adhere to new protocols. Moreover, public health was instrumental in developing isolation spaces for those infected.

Opportunity for Partnership

The pandemic created a deeper partnership between people experiencing homelessness and health workers, with each sector learning from the other. Adding health to the Tables allowed for discussions of homelessness to be understood as a public health issue because homelessness became compounded with other injustice issues (e.g., economic, social, and political) that directly affected this group's physical health, mental health and overall well-being while also triggering tremendous challenges for this group to access related health and social services. As noted by a service stakeholder: "I think there's more opportunities for more collaboration between Health and Housing … new opportunities for people to look at things differently." One of the critical findings of our study is the importance of partnerships. The two Tables signify the coming together of various organizations and players—some from the formal, government system, others from the informal, community, non-profit sector. Each system held key expertise and deliverables. Service stakeholders spoke eloquently of the importance of such collaborations and how the COVID-19 pandemic enabled deeper and more trusted relationships, such as "we are small enough that we built good relationships with each other, with folks on the ground, folks living in shelters." While these relations were seen as complicated at times, every participant spoke to a sense that the sector had become "more collaborative," "more collegial," involving vast learning spaces, knowledge sharing, and deeper trust. As noted above, having diverse lenses from diverse departments created a deeper understanding and learning of homelessness.

The importance of such collaboration was discussed by several participants who noted that trust was a key factor in the sectors' ability to mobilize and effectively roll out activities. It is important to note that one participant believed that the success of the sector in HRM had much to do with the partnerships and trust built over the past decade between individuals and organizations. Many collaborations between NGOs and community groups were established more than 10 years ago and these relationships were cultivated so that there was a foundation of partnerships that were well-developed and interconnected at the start of the pandemic. This foundation created a culture of trust among service sectors and PEHs, such that the addition of government and public health to these established relationships was met with acceptance and a sense of partnership. Moreover, the sector being small in scope (small province) also helped in creating more intimate collaborations and efficient and effective teamwork. Similar findings were identified in a study by Tebes et al. (2022) who created virtual and interactive Stress and Resilience Town Halls. These were accessible, scalable, and sustainable interventions to build mutual support, wellness, and resilience among healthcare workers within hospitals and health systems responding to emerging crises, pandemics, and natural disasters. The formation of these collaborations was instrumental in organizing a coordinated response during the COVID-19 pandemic. The benefits of which are now apparent and are seen as key to better supporting those who experience homelessness.

Non-government Organizations as Change Makers

While communication and sharing were key ingredients to how the sector responded to the pandemic, some participants also spoke to several important frustrations that were more prevalent in CBRM than HRM. To highlight, community non-profit organizations around the Tables were seen as the initiators of bringing partners together as they were "on the ground" and witnessing the shifting landscape. Communities were beginning to lockdown and important services and common spaces were beginning to close. These were extremely shocking and frightening times. All service stakeholders were deeply concerned about their individual and collective clientele, staff, families, and themselves. One of the authors speaks to this concern in a reflection article written during the first wave of the pandemic (see Karabanow, 2021). One service stakeholder expressed much guilt for "abandoning clients" when her service shut down. As the pandemic soared, there was a growing sense around the Tables that there was little leadership and little in terms of an initial action plan (other than several organizations having particular disaster guides/policies). This was indicated by a statement from one service stakeholder that "no plan was ready for this." As such, many members around the Tables believed that it was the local community organizations that stepped up and became the driving force of the response at first and that government was slow in action at times.

The importance of non-government organizations (NGOs) in leading during times of crisis has historical roots, a claim that is supported by organizational literature. Indeed, as identified by Sehgal (1991) during the AIDS pandemic, NGOs who had a long record of involvement in the field of health and social welfare, possessed several advantages over government agencies: 1) they had rich experience working at the community level; 2) their autonomous nature allowed them to respond more quickly; 3) they had access to marginalized groups; 4) they acted as a bridge between the community and the national level; 5) they often employed innovative methods; and 6) their method of operation allowed for cost-effectiveness. Research on the non-profit sector, homelessness, and COVID-19, as well as other disasters, has shown that non-profits are responsive and demonstrate leadership in service delivery vis-à-vis government, which overlap with the reasons identified by Sehgal (1991), including intimate knowledge of local populations and adaptability (Sundareswaran et al., 2015; Vickery, 2017). Our work supports the notion of NGOs as change makers during a time of crisis, further attesting to the necessity of these organizations.

It is important to recognize that the government was also innovative in its response to the COVID-19 pandemic with regards to homelessness. There is evidence in our study that some government officials redefined themselves as service providers to deal with the crisis. A good example was when government officials took on staffing roles at the emergency shelters (named "pop up shelters") set up to accommodate the reduced numbers of residents at existing shelters. However, linked to this notion is also the common sentiment among participants that the informal sector is rarely supported or praised by the government for their work. One service stakeholder noted that "shelter workers [and the sector in general] are the unsung heroes [of the pandemic]," yet they were late to be classified as essential workers and slow to receive personal protective equipment from the province. Therefore, greater recognition and support from the government is instrumental to the success of these organizations in managing a global crisis.

An Exhausted Sector

A significant, yet not surprising, theme of the study was that the homelessness sector is deeply strained and exhausted. One service stakeholder noted the significance of the "emotional, spiritual draining that like this pandemic has done to people who have been on the front lines." Service stakeholders described the system as "broken" and "in crisis." Moreover, the sector was overwhelmed prior to the COVID-19 pandemic and has been increasingly exhausted being the main frontline service delivery structure. While several stakeholders spoke of the system's strength in providing services during the early days of the crisis, others noted that there needs to be a system reinvention. The COVID-19 pandemic affected all sectors in the community, and frontline community organizations providing services to the homeless populations are to be counted as one of them. A service stakeholder summarized this sentiment by saying that:

> I think it's important that society ... come to the appreciation for what the non-profit sector does on a daily basis ... and when everybody is already exhausted and tapped out by normal circumstances, there's nothing left in the tank for crisis situations ... it's a sector that's highly under-resourced all the time. We've got to figure out a way to kind of rectify that situation.

Taken together, the housing service sector is already deeply strained, a situation that is only magnified by a crisis such as the COVID-19 pandemic.

Housing Security as a Social Determinant of Health

Coupled with this harsh reality of COVID-19 was the growing realization that NS (similar to many other provinces) was, and continues to, experience a housing affordability crisis (Canadian Center for Policy Alternatives, 2021; Roy et al., 2021; The NS Affordable Housing Commission, 2021). Many participants and service providers spoke of the tightening real estate market, the plethora of high-income development, the role of short-term vacation rentals, and a lack of investment in new rent geared to income units. Such a housing landscape increased the visibility of homelessness in the province. Not only were there more people living rough, looking for housing, turned away from shelters, or recently evicted, but there were also more discussions in public discourse (primarily in media) as to the vulnerability of this sector. Homelessness, poverty, and housing became overt issues in civil society. As one service stakeholder noted, "the problem has been so exposed it can't be ignored, nor should it."

The COVID-19 pandemic was a health disaster, and the public health responses to the crisis had to account for the significance of every sector in society. As such, with its spectrum of vulnerabilities and risks, homelessness became a grave concern to public health. While not always the case in the past, housing and poverty began to be viewed from a health perspective. A service stakeholder observed that:

> There is more focus on housing stability, there is more focus on harm reduction … there is more of an understanding of homelessness as a parcel of social determinants of health. It took a health crisis to put homelessness on the agenda again.

To manage the pandemic, we needed to embrace a wide array of social determinants of health, from ethnicity to geography to income to housing stability. While not a new paradigm within academia and service provision, the social determinant of health lens became embraced widely through civil society, so much so that the provincial government introduced a temporary rent cap and a temporary ban on evictions due to financial hardship as well as creating a task force to explore affordable housing (Province of NS, 2021). Just as the COVID-19 pandemic made everyone collectively vulnerable, the housing affordability crisis in NS reinforces this sentiment. It is no longer a single, ostracized community of individuals who are experiencing housing insecurity, but individuals who do not fit within the stereotypical view of being homeless. This change in narrative could be a driving force that puts housing security as a social determinant of health in the forefront of discussion, creating the potential for positive change for everyone experiencing or at risk of housing insecurity.

New Responses

An unexpected core finding from our study is that there are some outcrops to the pandemic that are significantly beneficial to the homelessness sector. As one participant experiencing homelessness noted: "It's almost a paradox, or an almost an irony, that in many ways, when I'm especially looking at it now … things seem to have improved in terms of what I have access to." With loss came some benefits. A prime example spoken to by most participants was that while there was a drastic reduction in services throughout the crisis (from shelter space to outreach services to access/availability of other supports), COVID-19 also forced existing services to restructure their provisions to be more health protective. All participants experiencing homelessness spoke to the fact that remodeled shelters were less crowded, provided more individual space, were cleaner, less violent, and more "dignified." Notwithstanding the grave loss of support when the province was in lockdown with a devastating toll on those in need, in order to follow public health guidelines and with financial infusions, services were able to create more compassionate spaces of care. A service stakeholder reported that "even the piece around creating the snugs [individual private spaces], that's a permanent change that the shelter will now be able to provide more dignified shelter … instead of being stacked up in bunk beds."

The addition of public health to the Tables discussions and the establishment of a deep collaboration between this agency and housing is another important outcome of the COVID-19 pandemic. Stakeholders have already experienced the benefits of this collaboration and are interested in deepening this relationship. The Tables also produced some significant responses to the pandemic, as described during interviews with service providers. In CBRM, public outdoor washrooms and "comfort sites" (with shower and laundry facilities) were created to provide for the physical and social needs of those experiencing homelessness (Doll et al., 2022). With the province in lockdown, these initiatives were crucial for those without access to washrooms and/or safe spaces to warm up, receive food, and connect with service providers.

In Halifax, hotels were used to house those on the street and/or in crowded shelters. Initially, hotels were used by the province to house couples and those with severe health issues. Soon after, several shelters moved their operations into hotels to provide their clientele with individual living arrangements during the pandemic. Later, hotel rooms were used for homeless individuals waiting for test results or quarantining. In Halifax, there was funding for renovations to existing shelters and supportive housing complexes to make these spaces adhere to public health ordinances (more individualized spacing, less numbers of residents, more hand washing stations, etc.). The majority of participants experiencing homelessness spoke highly of these new arrangements—speaking to how services were more "dignified," "less crowded," "more trauma informed," "safer," and "healthier" that helped them feel increased safety and less stress.

In Halifax, the provincial government took to frontline operations by setting up three "pop up shelters" to accommodate the reduction in bed numbers at existing shelters. While there were numerous critiques around the staffing, coordinating, training, and collective living arrangements within these sites, they did serve the purpose for allowing the existing shelters to reduce numbers. Halifax also saw a combined public health and community-based health clinic trial of a managed alcohol initiative that provided managed doses of alcohol to those experiencing homelessness and alcohol addiction. Last, a dedicated public health phone line was developed to support shelters in directing clients to testing, waiting, and quarantining spaces.

Discussion and Recommendations

All of the above initiatives worked, some better than others, but in the end, the creative, thoughtful, and quickly mobilized actions of service stakeholders supported the unique needs of homeless individuals and allowed some respite, safety, and shelter away from the pandemic. Many service stakeholders spoke about the unique opportunity that the COVID-19 pandemic presented in terms of being able to "think outside the box" and experiment with solutions. These thoughts were undoubtedly shaped by environments in which there were increased amounts of federal and provincial funding. The spread of the virus within the homeless communities was abated by quick actions of service providers to offer individual living spaces.

The hotel model works and provides a more dignified, healthy, quick, and efficient way to house individuals during a pandemic. As such, safe housing is the crucial element for such a disaster. Affordable, supportive, and sustainable housing has been lauded by housing experts as the only way forward. As one service stakeholder noted, "the legacy is a cultural shift to housing," while another service stakeholder noted that "the tone has changed" and housing is now the key focus. There were several articulations around the need to move some housing outside of the market economy (such as public and social housing for example) to make this a reality. Along these lines, one takeaway from the research is that there appears to be a deeper and more critical understanding of the complexity of housing and homelessness. As such, many participants noted that this research was important in order to script a "road map" as to what happened and to "document" the process in order to build "muscle memory" and support safety planning in the future. A short animated film, entitled *You Are Pretty Much On Your Own … The Two Disasters of Homelessness and The Pandemic*[1], was created by the research team as a way to disseminate broadly important findings that can lead to such a road map. This publicly available video converts the academic findings into an easily understandable format and serves as an educational tool to raise the general public's awareness regarding homelessness around them. This tool also informs stakeholders on how to improve their services and decision-making processes to better support this group.

Finally, it is extremely important to reemphasize that partnerships and collaboration are key and the most fundamental foundation to the pandemic response. All service stakeholders expressed notions of "needing each other," "not feeling alone," and "being trusted." Most importantly, the notion that such relationships and partnerships were the results of past decades of working together to build safe, trustworthy, and collegial landscapes was crucial. However, it is important to note that there was a lack of first voice representation (those experiencing homelessness) around these Tables; as such, many participants experiencing homelessness spoke of feeling uninformed and disconnected from important messaging.

Conclusion

The full spectrum of impacts of the COVID-19 pandemic has been and continues to be widespread throughout the globe. As the world reopens and enters the recovery stage, we are witnessing increased levels of anxiety, depression, loneliness, stress, and isolation alongside formal and informal health and social care systems that continue to be strained and overwhelmed. In the context of limited social and health service resources, homeless populations are a deeply marginalized segment of society that have weathered significant stress and neglect throughout the pandemic, during the recovery stage, and beyond. Taking care of the vulnerable and marginalized in disaster and non-disaster settings is vital to building just societies worldwide. Focusing on the COVID-19-specific interventions toward people experiencing homelessness in two communities in NS, this study illustrates evidence-based strategies to fulfill this group's needs, include PEH in advocating for their rights and reduce their vulnerabilities in the public health emergency response stage of COVID-19.

COVID-19 provides tremendous opportunities for different stakeholders to collaboratively understand the existing injustice in our societies and continually develop solutions to support vulnerable and marginalized populations. This study sheds light upon best practices and lessons from the field to include PEHs in deciding what actions are needed to ensure that they will not be forgotten in future disasters. The hope of this study is to raise awareness on the part of the general public and the public, private, and not-for-profit sectors to support not only people experiencing homelessness but other visible and invisible vulnerable and marginalized groups.

Note

1 <https://www.youtube.com/watch?v=qyVABjL55x8>

Bibliography

Canadian Center for Policy Alternatives. (2021). *Keys to a housing secure future for all Nova Scotians.* <https://policyalternatives.ca/publications/reports/keys-housing-secure-future-all-nova-scotians>

Corburn, J., Vlahov, D., Mberu, B., Riley, L., Caiaffa, W. T., Rashid, S. F., Ko, A., Patel, S., Jukur, S., Martínez-Herrera, E., Jayasinghe, S., Agarwal, S., Nguendo-Yongsi, B., Weru, J., Ouma, S., Edmundo, K., Oni, T., & Ayad, H. (2020). Slum health: Arresting COVID-19 and improving well-being in urban informal settlements. *Journal of Urban Health, 97*(3), 348–357. <https://doi.org/10.1007/S11524-020-00438-6>

Doll, K., Karabanow, J., Hughes, J., Leviten-Reid, C., & Wu, H. (2022). Homelessness within the COVID-19 pandemic in two Nova Scotian communities. *International Journal on Homelessness, 2*(1), 6–22. <https://doi.org/10.5206/IJOH.2022.1.14227>

Gaetz, S., Barr, C., Friesen, A., Harris, B., Hill, C., Kovacs-Burns, K., Pauly, B., Turner, A., & Morsolais, A. (2012). Canadian definition of homelessness. *Toronto: Canadian Observatory on Homelessness Press.*

Gin, J. L., Levine, C. A., Canavan, D., & Dobalian, A. (2022). Including Homeless Populations in Disaster Preparedness, Planning, and Response: A Toolkit for Practitioners. *Journal of Public Health Management and Practice, 28*(1), E62–E72. <https://doi.org/10.1097/PHH.0000000000001230>

Government of Canada, S. C. (2022, February 9). *Profile table, Census Profile, 2021 Census of Population—Nova Scotia [Province].* <https://www12.statcan.gc.ca/census-recensement/2021/dp-pd/prof/index.cfm?Lang=E>

Karabanow, J. (2006). Becoming a street kid: Exploring the stages of street life. *Journal of Human Behavior in the Social Environment, 13*(2), 49–72.

Karabanow, J. (2021). A reflection on living through COVID-19 as a social work professor. *Qualitative Social Work, 20*(1–2), 439–442.

Karabanow, J., Bozcam, E. S., Hughes, J., & Wu, H. (2022). Lessons learned: COVID 19 and individuals experiencing homelessness in the global context. *International Journal on Homelessness, 2*(1), 160–174.

Karabanow, J., Kidd, S., Frederick, T., & Hughes, J. (2018). *Homeless youth and the search for stability*. Wilfred Laurier University Press.

Karabanow, J., Wu, H., Doll, K., Leviten-Reid, C., & Hughes, J. (2023). Promoting emergency response for homeless service agencies: Field-based recommendations from two municipalities in Nova Scotia, Canada. *Natural Hazards Review, 24*(2), 06023001. <https://doi.org/10.1061/NHREFO.NHENG-1498>

Manthorpe, J., Cornes, M., O'Halloran, S., & Joly, L. (2015). Multiple exclusion homelessness: The preventive role of social work. *The British Journal of Social Work, 45*(2), 587–599. <https://doi.org/10.1093/bjsw/bct136>

Osborn, E., Every, D., & Richardson, J. (2019). Disaster preparedness: Services for people experiencing homelessness and the pressure-cooker response. *The Australian Journal of Emergency Management, 34*(1), 58–64.

Perri, M., Dosani, N., & Hwang, S. W. (2020). COVID-19 and people experiencing homelessness: Challenges and mitigation strategies. *CMAJ, 192*(26), E716–E719. <https://doi.org/10.1503/cmaj.200834>

Pixley, C. L., Henry, F. A., DeYoung, S. E., & Settembrino, M. R. (2022). The role of homelessness community based organizations during COVID-19. *Journal of Community Psychology, 50*(4), 1816–1830.

Province of Nova Scotia. (2020). Strengthening health system and new measures. News release. May 24. <https://novascotia.ca/news/release/?id=20200324003>

Ralli, M., Arcangeli, A., & Ercoli, L. (2021). Homelessness and COVID-19: Leaving no one behind. *Annals of Global Health, 87*(1), 1–3. <https://doi.org/10.5334/AOGH.3186>

Roy, L. C., Leviten-Reid, M., Digou, M., Gyorfi, J., MacQueen, J., & Gotell, C. (2021). *Service-based homelessness count 2021: Counting those experiencing homelessness in the Eastern Zone*. Cape Breton University, Nova Scotia Health. <https://www.endhomelessnesstoday.ca/images/Report_-_Service-Based_Homelessness_Count_for_Eastern_Nova_Scotia_2021.pdf>

Sehgal, P. N. (1991). Prevention and control of AIDS: The role of NGOs. *Health for the Millions, 17*(4), 31–33.

Service Nova Scotia and Internal Services. (2021, October 20). Amendments strengthen tenant protections and provide clarity for landlords. <https://novascotia.ca/news/release/?id=20211020004#:~:text=the%20current%20ban%20on%20evictions,of%20emergency%2C%20whichever%20is%20sooner>

Strauss, A., & Corbin, J. M. (1990). *Basics of qualitative research: Grounded theory procedures and techniques*. Sage Publications, Inc.

Sundareswaran, M., Ghazzawi, A., & O'Sullivan, T. L. (2015). Upstream disaster management to support people experiencing homelessness. *PLoS Currents, 7*, <https://doi.org/10.1371/currents.dis.95f6b76789ce910bae08b6dc1f252c7d>

Tebes, J. K., Awad, M. N., Connors, E. H., Fineberg, S. K., Gordon, D. M., Jordan, A., Kravitz, R., Li, L., Ponce, A. N., Prabhu, M., Rubman, S., Silva, M. A., Steinfeld, M., Tate, D. C., Xu, K., & Krystal, J. H. (2022). The stress and resilience town hall: A systems response to support the health workforce during COVID-19 and beyond. *General Hospital Psychiatry, 77*, 80–87. <https://doi.org/10.1016/j.genhosppsych.2022.04.009>

The Nova Scotia Affordable Housing Commission. (2021). *Charting a new course for affordable housing in Nova Scotia.* <https://beta.novascotia.ca/sites/default/files/documents/1-2679/charting-new-course-affordable-housing-nova-scotia-en.pdf>

Uppal, S. (2022). *A portrait of Canadians who have been homeless.* <https://www150.statcan.gc.ca/n1/en/pub/75-006-x/2022001/article/00002-eng.pdf?st=cqzOnzc0>

Vickery, J. (2017). *Every day is a disaster: Homelessness and the 2013 Colorado floods.* [Doctoral dissertation, University of Colorado].

Wu, H., & Karabanow, J. (2020). COVID-19 and beyond: Social work interventions for supporting homeless population. *International Social Work, 63*(6), 790–794. <https://doi.org/10.1177/0020872820949625>

Wu, H., Karabanow, J., & Hoddinott, T. (2022). Building emergency response capacity: Social workers' engagement in supporting homeless communities during COVID-19 in Halifax, Nova Scotia, Canada. *International Journal of Environmental Research and Public Health, 19, 12713.* <https://doi.org/10.3390/ijerph191912713>

You Are Pretty Much on Your Own … The Two Disasters of Homelessness and The Pandemic—YouTube. (n.d.). Retrieved May 26, 2023, from <https://www.youtube.com/watch?v=qyVABjL55x8&ab_channel=ShannonLong>

Zufferey, C., & Parkes, A. (2019). Family homelessness in regional and urban contexts: Service provider perspectives. *Journal of Rural Studies, 70,* 1–8. <https://doi.org/10.1016/j.jrurstud.2019.08.004>

· 2 ·

A REFLEXIVE ACCOUNT OF FACILITATING AN ONLINE STUDY OF THE PANDEMIC EXPERIENCES OF CANADIAN YOUTH USING CELLPHILMS

Grace Skahan, S. M. Hani Sadati,
Shannon Roy, and Claudia Mitchell

Introduction

Facilitating workshops in arts-based research is a practice that is shaped by the contexts of relationships, structures, and institutions, as Burkholder et al. (2022) asserted in their edited collection on facilitating community-based research. For researchers, paying attention to the process and the environment in which one is facilitating can help to make decisions which aim to "do good," that center ethical ways of relating, and which go beyond researcher reflexivity (Burkholder et al., 2022; LeBel, 2022). Many scholars who are committed to participatory methods have noted the importance of paying attention to process in the context of participatory research and of thinking critically about ethical questions beyond regulatory ethical frames required by academic institutions (De Lange, 2012; Guishard & Tuck, 2013; Hale, 2001, as cited in Mitchell et al. 2017; Tuck, 2009). But what happens when so much of the research process is happening online? What does it mean for researchers when the process of facilitation, which already entails constant evaluating, adjusting, responding to participants, and meeting them "where they are at, physically, politically, emotionally, and spiritually" (Burkholder et al., 2022, p. 11), is held in a virtual context? What opportunities and/or challenges do researchers face when practicing online facilitation, including during the COVID-19 pandemic?

This chapter builds on the growing body of critical work addressing online facilitation. Specifically, it explores the process of facilitating an online research study[1] with Canadian youth[2] about their experiences of the COVID-19 pandemic. While there is a growing body of literature on facilitation more generally in participatory and arts-based research (see Burkholder et al., 2022; Garcia et al., 2023; MacEntee et al., 2022; Vanner et al., 2022), online facilitation is becoming a mode of facilitation in and of itself. Using a qualitative, participatory, arts-based framework, we used *cellphilming methodology* (cellphone + film) to create a space for youth to express how they felt the pandemic impacted them, how they dealt with the challenges, what they would like teachers and policymakers to know, and what has given them hope during these times. Given what we were seeing in the early days of the pandemic in relation to school closures, we were particularly interested in what messages young people would have for teachers and professors, and youth-focused policy makers in areas such as education and mental health. Indeed, their cellphilms speak to the many stressors that youth were going through and demonstrate the need for critically thinking through online facilitation. We begin this chapter by providing context on online facilitation, the mental health and well-being of Canada's youth, and arts-based methods and cellphilming. We then provide some background on this research project and explore some salient themes which emerged in the cellphilms created by youth. To examine the process of facilitating an online study, we take a reflexive approach, offering reflections from Shannon, Claudia, and Hani, the three facilitators who were present during the data collection workshops. We finish this chapter by discussing lessons learned about facilitating online and youth's mental health.

Online Facilitation

Many research projects that were intended to be carried out in person transitioned to online beginning in March 2020. Although the scholarly work that addresses the methodological and ethical questions around this transition is limited, research on online facilitation and online support groups can offer some starting points for discussing our experience of facilitating research with young people during the pandemic and offers an understanding of what changes when groups shift from being in person to online. The disembodied environment of being in groups online poses significant obstacles to the ways people emotionally regulate each other and eye contact with participants and co-leaders (or co-facilitators) is lost (Weinberg, 2020). The limited view (e.g., only their head shot or sometimes no video at all) can also make it more difficult to understand how group members are feeling (Parks, 2020). The additional context of body language and in-person interactions that often helps us understand what others are saying is missing online.

In the literature on conducting participatory research online, some challenges noted include a lack of researcher control, difficulty in engaging some participants in online discussions, difficulty in creating/maintaining equity and rapport, a lack of privacy, and a lack of confidentiality in group settings (Dodds & Hess, 2020; Hall et al., 2021). In their research on youth alcohol consumption during the pandemic, Dodds and Hess (2020) further identified a lack of non-verbal communication and inadequate physical set up given that tablets and computers do not always provide an optimal view.

According to Dodds and Hess (2020), some advantages of online participatory research include the participants being comfortable, feeling safe, enjoying participating from home, and being familiar with communicating online. In terms of best practices, when conducting focus groups online, smaller groups of under five people are often favored (Lobe & Morgan, 2021; Lobe et al., 2020). In the context of conducting research online during a stressful time such as a pandemic, Hall et al. (2021) also noted the value of using creative or therapeutic methods that benefit participants given that asking people to participate in research projects during a pandemic has an added ethical complication since people are already generally distressed.

Canadian Youth's Mental Health and Well-being

Early estimations from the United Nations predicted that youth would be the most affected by the pandemic because of the impact it has had during important moments of their development (UNICEF, 2020). In research on the mental health of youth living in Canada, some salient issues that have emerged since the beginning of the pandemic include depression (Craig et al., 2020; Stewart et al., 2022), anxiety (Birnie et al., 2022; Craig et al., 2020; Stewart et al., 2022), eating disorders (Agostino et al., 2021; Singh et al., 2022), and substance use (Chaiton et al., 2022; Salmon et al., 2022; Sheikhan et al., 2022). These studies also show that trends often differ along demographic lines such as gender, disabilities, race, and sexuality.

Apart from an uptick in mental health issues, Canadian youth have also experienced more physical health issues and significant barriers related to work and housing (Abramovich et al., 2022; Arbour-Nicitopoulos, 2022; Caldwell et al., 2022; Lannoy et al., 2022; Lindsay & Ahmed, 2022; Noble et al., 2022). There may also be lingering impacts of the pandemic on youth, related to their mental health, housing situation, and substance use (Hawke et al., 2021; Noble et al., 2022; Salmon et al., 2022). For these reasons, gaining a better understanding of Canadian youth's experiences with the pandemic, while conducting ethical research that considers youth's vulnerable state of well-being, continues to be of utmost importance.

Although what were considered perhaps the most critical stages of the pandemic have now passed, COVID-19 persists, as do its ramifications.

Methods

The research presented in this chapter is part of a project that aimed to gain a better understanding of Canadian youth's experiences of the COVID-19 pandemic. We conceived of this project at the very beginning of the pandemic in April 2020 and therefore, we did not have to adjust our research methods given that we planned the project with the understanding that there would likely be some degree of physical restrictions in place when we arrived at the data collection phase. Arts-based methods have been hailed by many as a transformative way to do research. Given the therapeutic dimension of arts-based research, various scholars have noted the benefits of these methods as an alternative and more suitable approach for doing research during a time of enhanced stress and vulnerability, such as the COVID-19 pandemic (Hall et al., 2021; Liegghio & Caragata, 2021).

To approach the exploration of young people's experiences during the pandemic, we used an arts-based method called cellphilming. *Cellphilm*, a term coined by Dockney and Tomaselli (2009), is a combination of the words cellphone and film. This technique uses the cellphone (or other devices), an object that most people are familiar with and carry around all the time. The videos created with this technique are usually short in length (one to three minutes) and aim to address a particular social issue (MacEntee et al., 2016). As highlighted by Mitchell et al. (2016), cellphilms help bridge the gap between an "insider" and an "outsider" in participatory research because cellphilm techniques make use of technology (i.e., cellphones) that participants are already familiar with. Bridging this gap was important for this research, especially in the context of doing research with youth "at a distance" during a time of heightened vulnerability.

In the data that we report on here, there were a total of 33 young people between the ages of 16 and 24 from across Canada. Participants were recruited by contacting organizations across Canada who work with youth, through word of mouth, and by advertising on social media. Participants received a 50$ Amazon gift card as compensation for their participation. In order to receive the link for the first workshop, participants needed to fill out a consent form. This process ensured that we did not accidentally record someone who had not consented to participating in the study, given that the workshops were audio recorded.

Participation in this project included two one-hour data collection workshops, both of which were conducted online via Zoom. These workshops involved two to three researchers as facilitators and two to eight young people. While most workshops were conducted in English, two of them were conducted in French. The audio recordings of the workshops, which were later transcribed verbatim, comprise the data analyzed in this chapter along with the reflections by each facilitator.

The first of the two workshops was an overview of the research project and how to make a cellphilm. In that workshop, we provided participants with the prompt: "How have you felt the pandemic has impacted you, how have you dealt with the arisen challenges, and what would you like teachers and policymakers to know?" We altered this prompt slightly in later workshops, asking participants to consider what could help them move forward and what would give them hope. We want to draw particular attention to this change in wording in recognition of what we saw as a particularly challenging time for many of the participants. Most of the online workshops we are reporting on here took place between December 2021 and March 2022, a time that coincided with resurgence in the number of COVID-19 cases in many parts of Canada as a result of the Omicron variant.

During the second workshop, each participant was invited to introduce their cellphilm by speaking briefly about it. One of the facilitators, who had received all the cellphilms from youth prior to the workshop, then shared their screen and we watched the cellphilm created. After all the cellphilms had been screened, participants were invited to discuss questions such as: What do you see as the key themes? Did you learn something that surprised you? Are there themes you thought you would see but didn't? What do you think these cellphilms say? Do you think they speak to any particular audience such as policy makers, professors, administrators or other? What changes are the cellphilms calling for?

Findings

We divide the data[3] from the cellphilming workshops conducted with youth in two parts. In part one, we offer an overview of key themes raised by the youth during the workshops, where mental health issues were key. In part two, the three facilitators, Shannon, Claudia, and Hani, reflect on the facilitation process.

Part One: Key Themes from the Workshops

Our analysis revealed several key themes about youth experiences during the pandemic and revealed much about how youth felt about participating in a research project of this kind. Questions of youth's mental health and discussions related to mental illness, exhaustion related to being online, losses, stress, and racism frequently dominated the workshops. These issues often intersected with one another. Some youth also spoke to the positive dimensions of health and well-being related to their pandemic experiences. During the workshops, a recurring theme that was identified was related to the experience itself of participating in a study on the pandemic. Participants spoke about the vulnerability they felt in sharing personal stories in a group setting as well as the therapeutic and healing dimension of articulating their thoughts and feelings related to their pandemic experiences.

Youth Experiences with the COVID-19 Pandemic

Mental Health Struggles. In describing their lived experiences during the pandemic, many participants talked about mental health challenges stemming from the government-enforced distancing restrictions. This was a recurring theme in the cellphilms and also in the screening workshop discussions. Participants mentioned struggles such as depression, insomnia, and anxiety. During one of the screening sessions, one participant noted that, "a main theme that is seen [in the cellphilms] is depression and also anxiety for many people. And also the fear of the unknown is literally displayed in almost all the cellphilms." Various participants also named social anxiety as such, and another participant described it as follows:

> And it's something that I'm still kind of unlearning—feeling comfortable around people in groups now that we're allowed to gather again. And it's also made me kind of overthink social interactions. I feel like, you know, I'm not used to being with people in an intimate context, like inside my house, like I get—I'm already someone who's quite introverted and reserved to begin with. So it's interesting how now being put in these social contexts, I'm way more introspective and I think more self-conscious than I've ever been before. Because it's as if, like, we haven't done this in a long time. And so, you know, you just kind of learned to be on your own.

Social anxiety was a recurring challenge that youth mentioned, which was made worse by physical distancing and the lack of interaction that has characterized so many people's lives during the pandemic.

Online Exhaustion and Losses. Youth talked about the difficulty of school, socializing, and/or volunteering commitments all being online. The pandemic sometimes also led to young people doing their research-related field work, first internships, or first professional experiences online. Many spoke to a sense of loss stemming from pandemic restrictions, and about grieving this important time in their life when they are entering adulthood and are supposed to be exploring their potential, discovering who they are, furthering themselves in school and their careers, and having new experiences, as opposed to living through their screens.

Stress. Youth often spoke about juggling multiple commitments during the COVID-19 pandemic. They spoke about stress related to schoolwork, employment, social pressures, and sometimes the additional responsibilities of taking care of siblings or assisting their families with household chores. They also spoke of the limited space and privacy within homes.

Racism. Adding to the heightened stress were issues related to racism. For example, some youth talked about the increased racism toward Asian people. Another youth spoke of the elevated visibility and discussions around race more generally, initiated by the murder of George Floyd. This young person said:

> Also with the polarizing point, I remember, it was in 2020 when the whole like, Black Lives Matter movement really picked up speed, because of all the stuff that was happening. And I remember that was in June and I'm part of the Black community, and I remember how mentally exhausted I was from a pandemic. And then, obviously, it was happening and also having to write like final exams online and try to—I don't think I've ever experienced the mental exhaustion and like, even the emotional exhaustion, and how difficult it was just to try to like grapple with everything, even within myself just to like, reflect I don't even think I wanted to reflect on anything.

This passage demonstrates the accumulation of stress, and how compounding factors such as racial inequity made it difficult for youth to process what was happening.

Positive Experiences of Well-Being. Some youth also spoke of the positive impacts that having so much time alone during the pandemic had on them. Time alone led to discovering unexpected interests, exploring new hobbies, or reconsidering career paths. In one of the cellphilm screening sessions, one youth talked about finding the entire pandemic experience fascinating. In the context of talking about the cellphilm they made, they said:

> But I was really interested by the vaccine and the whole process of COVID. And what we had to go through, so I decided to do community work with my friends. And we actually have a podcast about a vaccine that we're doing, which allowed us to talk to many professional, professional health workers and stuff to interview them about the vaccine under their experience.

For this youth, the novel and unprecedented dimension of the pandemic itself prompted a new and generative project that helped them cope with pandemic-related stress.

A number of youth also spoke about how the pandemic-related physical distancing and isolation requirements led them to spend more time with their families which they appreciated. Though there was a dominant theme of difficulties related to mental health and well-being in the screening sessions and cellphilms, some youth made it clear that while they recognized a general state of struggle among youth, they personally did not have that experience. In some cases, they felt the experience led to positive outcomes.

Youth Experiences of Participating in the Study

Vulnerability in Participation. Participating in this research was often not a neutral experience for participants, which they shared with facilitators and other participants. In some cases, youth expressed being uncomfortable sharing their personal stories in front of a group of people whom they most often did not know and in some cases could not even see or hear because of cameras and microphones being off. While as facilitators we sensed this, sometimes by a lack of participation, this discomfort was also sometimes explicitly shared. For example, one youth articulated this by saying, "I do find it hard just to throw in some of my random experiences. Not random, but my experiences to just a group, if you like, black boxes right now. Or it's like, some of my personal experiences are pretty intense." This comment demonstrates an important question and source of concern for facilitators. Perhaps relatedly, some of the smallest workshops, which consisted of only two participants, were found to be the richest. Participants shared more and appeared to be more comfortable.

A Therapeutic Dimension. While participation in this project was sometimes evidently challenging and uncomfortable for participants, there seemed at times to be a therapeutic dimension to hearing about others' stories and sharing their own. Some said participating helped them feel less alone because in watching other people's cellphilms, they realized they shared similar experiences with other young people living in Canada. They talked about how hearing stories like theirs was reassuring and helped them better understand things about themselves or their own experiences.

When participants shared cellphilms containing particularly difficult subject matter, group members offered consolation, support, or words of encouragement either directly or in the chat. Some participants spoke about the therapeutic dimension of the process of creating the cellphilm, since it motivated them to actively process and think about their experiences of the past few years. Some also mentioned that the process of creating the cellphilms boosted their confidence in their public speaking and creative skills.

Part Two: Reflections from Facilitators

Reflective practice is an essential element in the development and growth of educators. Hence, each of the facilitators of the workshops has shared a brief reflection of their experience facilitating online workshops with youth that look to best practices in this educational space. Schön (1983) explains that reflection can be defined as thinking of an experience as it happens or pondering it after it has taken place. By engaging in reflective practice, educators and facilitators can analyze their strategies, evaluate their effectiveness, and make adjustments, leading to continuous improvement. Furthermore, through continuous reflective practice, educators and facilitators can build professional knowledge, skills, and competencies that inform effective pedagogical practices (Schön, 1983). In our reflections, we look at questions such as, what actions supported engaging dialogue among participants? Were there moments when the participants expressed a need for us as facilitators to make them more comfortable in that space? What did we notice about how youth engaged with each other in the online workshops, and how did our practice evolve over time and why?

The following reflections are meant to offer insights into the facilitation process itself, highlighting some of the tensions and challenges in this work.

Shannon

I came into the Canadian Youth Talking About Pandemic Experiences (CYTAPE) as a first-year Ph.D. student. While I was new to cellphilming and conducting online workshops, I had been a teacher for 12 years, which offered me practical knowledge and skills for how to facilitate educational experiences with youth. Being a practicing artist, I brought lenses of aesthetics and creativity to the workshops.

As a research group, we took time after each workshop to discuss and reflect on how the workshop had unfolded. During this time, we often came to new realizations and wished to make minor (or sometimes more significant) adjustments to our next workshop. Elements such as including space for participants to give a brief introduction to their cellphilm before starting and including a question about participants' creative choices were examples of mindful additions. We noted these specific adjustments because they were the most significant changes that we made throughout the process that allowed our participants to expand on their pandemic experiences. Each new inclusion in our process improved the quality of our workshop in terms of the richness of our discussions. Throughout the process, I began to see cellphilms as a true form of art, and while I knew that going in, the creativity I saw coming out of our workshops showed me that cellphilm creators and participants were real artists.

Some of our workshops resulted in lots of detailed information about participants, and other workshop dynamics were more reserved discussions where the information provided by the participants was more straightforward. I continued to reflect on how to get a great depth of discussion during each and every workshop with participants, ultimately realizing that there is no perfect way to conduct every workshop. Working with a unique group of individuals every second workshop made it nearly impossible to know how to facilitate that group of people flawlessly. As I often saw when I was working in the classroom, each workshop was a new and unique experience comprised of endless variables—many uncontrollable from our end. For example, we were not able to control how forthcoming with information each participant would be, or even if they would decide to turn on their camera so we could see facial expressions. Still, we reflected regularly to create a safe space that was valuable for the participants and brought forth rich data for the project.

The most challenging component of facilitating these workshops for me was being unable to see everyone's face while conducting the workshop. As a teacher, I rely heavily on my senses, particularly watching my student's body language and expressions to guide my teaching and know when to adjust, add, or eliminate bits of information to tailor a lesson to students' needs and achieve ultimate engagement. Teaching to a blank screen is highly challenging, and most of the time, our participants would have their cameras turned off. Understandably, many youth wanted to remain private or have a more confidential experience. Still, as a facilitator, I found this difficult. I wanted to engage the participants, and reading the room is part of how I best engage my students. MacEntee et al. (2016) stated, "during presentations and screening events, my eyes are on the audience. Are they following the narrative? Can they follow what is being said? Maybe it is too loud?" (p. 149). This statement resonated with me as I would follow a similar thought process during an in-person screening; however, the wealth of these intuitive education practices is not all available to us teaching black boxes on a screen. What this taught me was that it was even more imperative to ensure a comfortable space for participants when online.

The lack of non-verbal cues in online communication can create a sense of distance and reduce the emotional intensity of sharing personal information. To mitigate this, we found that allowing people to take their time to think about their responses allowed more responses to come through. Additionally, letting participants know that we would give them space and time to share was helpful so that awkward silences were less of a concern. We also informed participants that they could share at their comfort level and that they need not feel pressured to share anything they did not want to. These factors created a more comfortable and safer environment where people could open up and share their personal experiences online.

Claudia

When we started the online workshops, I do not think I had fully imagined what it would be like to convene a group of strangers on an online platform about a topic like the pandemic, and where people were required to screen their cellphilm productions. I was no stranger to online teaching, and of course there are inevitably pedagogical hiccups and gaffs. My questions may fall flat. Conversations may be happening in the chat, and I miss some. Establishing some sort of process is key, but so is some sort of rapport. Somehow in setting up these workshops with sometimes as few as two or three people—and most at five or six—these same limitations apply. In some ways, it was like having a "first class" over and over and over again, where we worked hard to build rapport and provide a space for people to feel comfortable to participate.

Who signs up to share their experiences of the pandemic? We were offering a small financial compensation, so I doubt that would be the driving factor. When asked, some people said they were intrigued by the idea of learning something new or doing something creative. But the part that was the most challenging was the idea of what people were addressing and revealing in their cellphilms: feeling isolated, cut off from friends, locked in with family. One person talked about just staying in her bedroom for weeks on end and so her bedroom was also the setting for her cellphilm. Many of these narratives were very moving, and they were even more so when people spoke about the "story behind the story." It finally dawned on us that this was not just about online facilitation of a process of making cellphilms. It was more of a recognition that this work, in and of itself, was much more in the category of mental health support. What preparation did we have to do this? What preparation is needed?

And then there is timing. Because of starting the interviews in December 2021, some participants were dealing with the newer strains of Omicron and were social distancing again, even though they had been relatively free of COVID-19 for some time. We often wondered whether our questions about the pandemic should be in the past, the present, or the future. And this varied from one region to another in Canada, as well as from one participant's experiences to others.

Hani

I have participated in and presented webinars, online workshops, courses, and conferences. The difference in the CYTAPE project was that it was the first time I conducted research online to collect data. In all my previous online events, the primary goal was either knowledge dissemination, awareness creation, idea exchange, or contributing to collective action. But in CYTAPE, the primary goal was to collect as much reliable data as possible. The workshops were organized so all phases could contribute to addressing the main research questions. Although this data collection process might be similar in in-person cellphilming research, the restrictions of online space made it more challenging and potential issues arising from being online added stress sometimes. For example, any technical issue (e.g., interruption in internet connection) that disconnect either the researcher or the participant from the workshop could stop or affect the data collection process. Or conversations with participants while their videos were off could erode the opportunity for researchers to have body language or facial expressions as complementary to verbal communication.

It is understandable when participants who are strangers to each other are in a virtual room, they might be concerned about showing their faces and revealing their identities, particularly when they express deep personal experiences. In our workshops, some participants decided to keep their videos off. Although, from my perspective, this anonymity created a more comfortable space for sharing thoughts, it also made it challenging for researchers to recognize the participants' identities to ensure the person belongs to the research's target population. To address this challenge, at the beginning of each session and during the short icebreaking activities we informally asked participants some questions to learn more about their location (such as what the weather is like, how their school is, or the name of their city). The answers to these inquiries served as indicators to help researchers verify participants' identities.

When conducting online research, researchers do not have the same opportunity or amount of time to interact with participants and establish a solid participant-facilitator relationship, as they do in in-person research. For both parties, all prior information they have from each other is through a few email exchanges. So, in most cases, it is like someone pops up on a screen for one hour and then pops out! As a researcher with experience conducting in-person interviews and focus group discussions, I found that the researcher-participant relationship in CYTAPE was quite delicate since the entire pre-facilitation, facilitation, and post-facilitation process happened online. This delicacy did not necessarily affect the reliability of collected data, but it affected the immersivity and engagement of the research process. Overall, my experience of facilitating in the CYTAPE project showed that online facilitation helped create an environment where participants had the option to maintain their anonymity, which contributed to creating a psychologically safe space for our participants to speak out and freely share their pandemic experiences. At the same time, this form of facilitation also presented challenges that warrant further investigation particularly in the context of the personal experiences of young people.

Conducting the entire research project online had advantages, such as being time- and cost-effective, but it also came with some risks and uncertainties. In one instance, a participant unintentionally deleted their cellphilm from YouTube after the workshops had concluded. As a result, researchers were unable to access that cellphilm as a piece of data. Fortunately, since all the sessions were recorded (with the participants' consent), that particular cellphilm could be retrieved from the recorded session as it was screened during the workshop. As another example, in online workshops, I often had the stress of forgetting to press the record button, which could result in missing some parts of the data. While only a technical detail, it puts an extra psychological burden on the researcher's shoulders.

Indeed, while our concern of course was with the youth themselves, I also wanted to draw attention to the importance of considering the mental health of researchers, especially in online research facilitation. Although the mental health of researchers is equally important in both in-person and online facilitation processes, my experience in CYTAPE revealed to me that the latter comes with its own unique set of challenges that can exacerbate existing stressors or create new ones. As noted above, online research facilitators may face technological difficulties, such as software malfunctions, which can create additional pressure and frustration. Moreover, virtual communication may not be as effective in building rapport and trust with participants as face-to-face interactions, adding to the mental load of the facilitator. Given the pivotal role that research facilitators play in the success of a project, it is essential to acknowledge the potential impact of these challenges on their well-being.

Discussion

In conducting this study, we furthered our own understanding of promising practices for online facilitation and came away with a better understanding of concrete techniques that can support young people's well-being when engaging them in the co-production of knowledge.

In line with what previous researchers have noted (Lobe & Morgan, 2021; Lobe et al., 2020), a small group size of four or less led to more intimate sharing and seemed to ease participation and communication. Looking back on our earlier discussion of the limits of online groups (Dodds & Hess, 2020; Parks, 2020), our research showed us that communication barriers are indeed a significant challenge when online. Asking participants to introduce their cellphilm before showing it provided helpful context for everyone and helped make up for the lack of non-verbal communication. In this way, using multiple mediums for transmitting and discussing messages in the cellphilms (the cellphilm itself, the cellphilmmaker's explanation, and a couple of sentences shared on a PowerPoint about what the cellphilm is about) can help ensure everyone is following the discussion. This is a useful lesson that can perhaps be applied when facilitating arts-based workshops beyond the realm of cellphilming, and when trying to engage young people in a group discussion online.

Another promising practice we noted was the importance of attention to detail in the initial planning and coordination of our study, providing asynchronous material, and carefully considering the structure of the outreach and post-workshop stages. These are measures we put in place to varying degrees throughout this process to ease the burden of participating in a research project. We would repeat these measures again as participants seemed to appreciate them.

Easing the burden of participation was important due to the ethical dimension of asking those already under stress to participate in a project like this one (Hall et al. 2021). The stress that youth were under was brought up often in the discussions about their cellphilms. Issues such as mental illness, exhaustion related to being online, losses, and racism surfaced. In the future, in terms of outreach structure, we would put more emphasis on the distressing emotions that participation may surface. As noted in the findings, despite getting informed consent from participants, it at times appeared as though they did not realize how participating might raise difficult and uncomfortable feelings and might require more emotional effort than they had expected. Going forward, during the consent process, we would make an effort to explicitly mention that participation may be emotionally challenging and more stressful than expected, given the subject of the research, the general challenging atmosphere of the pandemic, and any other personal issues they may be experiencing.

An important tension to explore further is that between building trust and an intimate space for collaborating while also not forcing vulnerability on participants. It is vital to respect the privacy of young people and their agency to not turn their cameras on, even if at times this could have been an inhibitor to forming trust and a sense of connection, which is important for creating the conditions where people can feel comfortable being vulnerable by sharing their stories. Participants' choices to not put their cameras on, to not share their cellphilms, to not create a cellphilm at all, or to not answer our questions during the workshops were legitimate and of utmost importance to listen to. Conducting ethical research means respecting these choices and ensuring participants know that they have the choice to not participate at every moment. Drawing on theories of non-participation (Switzer, 2020; Tuck & Yang, 2014; Weaver et al., 2022), this decision to not participate should not be understood as necessarily something negative and can be interpreted as an act of youth agency or resistance. Respecting non-participation and/or different forms or extents of participation is an important lesson from this research that extends to post-pandemic contexts as well.

Young people's experiences of the pandemic and of taking part in our study point to some important takeaways and areas for future research for facilitating research online. The value of arts-based methods in an online study during a stressful time merits being further explored. Making cellphilms appeared to have had a positive and therapeutic effect for some due to the ease with which it helped participants express themselves about difficult topics and possibly reduced the stress of participation. Furthermore, some young people noted enjoying sharing their experiences with others and benefiting from hearing others' experiences. These results highlight the usefulness of an arts-based method like cellphilming in the context of a crisis like the COVID-19 pandemic and echo what other researchers have said on this topic (Hall et al., 2021; Liegghio & Caragata, 2021). It also aligns with what previous researchers have noted before and beyond the pandemic context concerning the positive and therapeutic values of arts-based methods (Fraser & al Sayah, 2011; Nowicka-Sauer, 2007).

Conclusion

With the onset of the COVID-19 pandemic, researchers sought new ways to create knowledge, given the many constraints that the pandemic generated. All research that has been conducted during the pandemic is in some ways about the pandemic, yet not all of it interrogates the pandemic's impact. While research continued to emerge during the pandemic about young people's experiences, little research has thus far addressed in depth the complexities of carrying out such research online. For this study, we used cellphilming to explore young people's experiences during the pandemic, and it became very clear that a great number of youth were dealing with stress and were exhausted from being online. Participating in a research project might have added stress because of the additional time they were being asked to spend online and because of their vulnerability. However, it was clear that in some workshops, participating in this project provided a much-needed source of connection. It provided an opportunity to process experiences in a group setting. These findings hold important weight for the role of facilitators. Some important takeaways for us as researchers and facilitators include the value of arts-based methods to ease participating in an online study during a stressful time and the importance of respecting youth's non-participation. We also furthered our own understanding of online facilitating. Some takeaways are the significance of creating a warm and welcoming space, the importance of detailed planning and coordinating, and the value of a small group. All of these findings, while especially important given the weight of living through a pandemic, are important considerations for conducting research that is mindful of youth's mental health more broadly beyond the context of a global crisis.

Notes

1 Funded by Quebec's Ministère de la Santé et des Services sociaux, the project is titled Young People, Well-being, and Connectedness in the Time of Distancing (later changed Canadian Youth Talking About Pandemic Experiences (CTYAPE). It contributes to illuminating the experiences, challenges, motivations, and stories of young people residing in Canada during and after the COVID-19 pandemic.
2 This study included youth residing in Canada regardless of their legal status.
3 In the period analyzed in this chapter, 26 cellphilms of 1–2 minutes were created (some of the 33 youth worked in small groups).

Bibliography

Abramovich, A., Pang, N., & Moss, A. (2022). Experiences of family violence among 2SLGBTQ+ youth at risk of, and experiencing, homelessness before and during the COVID-19 pandemic. *Journal of Gay & Lesbian Mental Health*, 1–24. <https://doi.org/10.1080/19359705.2022.2076759>

Agostino, H., Burstein, B., Moubayed, D., Taddeo, D., Grady, R., Vyver, E., Dimitropoulos, G., Dominic, A., & Coelho, J. S. (2021). Trends in the incidence of new-onset anorexia nervosa and atypical anorexia nervosa among youth during the COVID-19 pandemic in Canada. *JAMA network open*, 4(12), Article e2137395-e2137395. <https://doi:10.1001/jamanetworkopen.2021.37395>

Arbour-Nicitopoulos, K. P., James, M. E., Moore, S. A., Sharma, R., & Martin Ginis, K. A. (2022). Movement behaviours and health of children and youth with disabilities: Impact of the 2020 COVID-19 pandemic. *Paediatrics & Child Health*, 27(Supplement_1), S66–S71. <https://doi.org/10.1093/pch/pxac007>

Birnie, K. A., Kopala-Sibley, D. C., Pavlova, M., Nania, C. G., Bernier, E., Stinson, J. N., & Noel, M. (2022). The impact of the COVID-19 pandemic on youth with chronic pain and their parents: A longitudinal examination of who are most at risk. *Children*, 9(5), 745. <https://doi.org/10.3390/children9050745>

Burkholder, C., Aledebi, J. & Schwab-Cartas, J. (Eds.). (2022). *Leading and listening to community: Facilitating qualitative, arts-based & visual research for social change*. Routledge.

Caldwell, H. A., Faulkner, G., Tremblay, M. S., Rhodes, R. E., de Lannoy, L., Kirk, S. F., Rehman, L. & Moore, S. A. (2022). Regional differences in movement behaviours of children and youth during the second wave of the COVID-19 pandemic in Canada: Follow-up from a national study. *Canadian Journal of Public Health*, 113(4), 535–546. <https://doi.org/10.17269/s41997-022-00644-6>

Chaiton, M., Dubray, J., Kundu, A., & Schwartz, R. (2022). Perceived impact of COVID on smoking, vaping, alcohol and cannabis use among youth and youth adults in Canada. *The Canadian Journal of Psychiatry*, 67(5), 407–409.

Craig, S. G., Ames, M. E., Bondi, B. C., & Pepler, D. J. (2022). Canadian adolescents' mental health and substance use during the COVID-19 pandemic: Associations with COVID-19 stressors. *Canadian Journal of Behavioural Science/Revue canadienne des sciences du comportement 55*(1), 46. <https://doi.org/10.1037/cbs0000305>

De Lange, N. (2012). Researching to make a difference: Possibilities for social science research in the age of AIDS. *SAHARA-J: Journal of Social Aspects of HIV/AIDS, 9*, 3–10.

Dockney, J., & Tomaselli, K. G. (2009). Fit for the small (er) screen: Films, mobile TV and the new individual television experience. *Journal of African Cinema, 1*(1), 126–132.

Dodds, S., & Hess, A. C. (2020). Adapting research methodology during COVID-19: lessons for transformative service research. *Journal of Service Management, 32*(2), 203–217

Fraser, K. D., & Al Sayah, F. (2011). Arts-based methods in health research: A systematic review of the literature. *Arts & Health, 3*(2), 110–145.

Garcia, C. K., Mitchell, C., & Ezcurra, M. (2023). Not just any toolkit! What's facilitation got to do with it? In S. Shariff & C. Dietzel (Eds.), *IMPACTS: Reclaiming the role of universities to address sexual violence through multi-sector partnerships in law, arts and social media.* (pp. 147–174). Peter Lang.

Guishard, M., & Tuck, E. (2013). Youth resistance research methods and ethical challenges. In Guishard, M., & Tuck, E (Eds.), *Youth resistance research and theories of change* (pp. 193–206). Routledge.

Hale, C. R. (2001). What is activist research? *Social Science Research Council, 2*(1–2), 13–15.

Hall, J., Gaved, M., & Sargent, J. (2021). Participatory research approaches in times of Covid-19: A narrative literature review. *International Journal of Qualitative Methods, 20.* <https://doi.org/10.1177/16094069211010087>

Hawke, L. D., Szatmari, P., Cleverley, K., Courtney, D., Cheung, A., Voineskos, A. N., & Henderson, J. (2021). Youth in a pandemic: A longitudinal examination of youth mental health and substance use concerns during COVID-19. *BMJ open, 11*(10), Article e049209. <http://dx.doi.org/10.1136/bmjopen-2021-049209>

Lannoy, L., MacDonald, L., Barbeau, K., & Tremblay, M. S. (2022). Environmental scan of child and youth outdoor play-based projects, programs, activities and services available in Canada during the COVID-19 pandemic. *Children, Youth and Environments 32*(1), 84–127. <https://doi.org/10.1353/cye.2022.0004.>

LeBel, S. (2022). Facilitating queer art in the climate crisis. In Burkholder, C., Aledebi, J. & Schwab-Cartas, J. (Eds.). (2022). *Leading and listening to community: Facilitating qualitative, arts-based & visual research for social change.* Routledge.

Liegghio, M., & Caragata, L. (2021). COVID-19 and youth living in poverty: The ethical considerations of moving from in-person interviews to a photovoice using remote methods. *Affilia, 36*(2), 149–155.

Lindsay, S., & Ahmed, H. (2022). Barriers to school and work transitions for youth with and without a disability during the COVID-19 pandemic: A qualitative comparison. *Archives of Physical Medicine and Rehabilitation, 103*(3), Article e11-e12. https://doi.org/10.1016/j.apmr.2022.01.030

Lobe, B., Morgan, D., & Hoffman, K. A. (2020). Qualitative data collection in an era of social distancing. *International Journal of Qualitative Methods, 19.* <https://doi.org/10.1177/1609406920937875>

Lobe, B., & Morgan, D. L. (2021). Assessing the effectiveness of video-based interviewing: A systematic comparison of video-conferencing based dyadic interviews and focus groups. *International Journal of Social Research Methodology, 24*(3), 301–312.

MacEntee, K., Burkholder, C., & Schwab-Cartas, J. (Eds.). (2016). *What's a cellphilm?: Integrating mobile phone technology into participatory visual research and activism.* Sense. <https://doi.org/10.1007/978-94-6300-573-9>

MacEntee, K., Nyariro, M., Thompson, J., & Mitchell, C. (2022). A reflexive account of performing facilitation in participatory visual research for social change. In C. Burkholder, J. Aledebi, & J. Schwab-Cartas (Eds.). *Leading and listening to community: Facilitating qualitative, arts-based & visual research for social change.* Routledge.

Mitchell, C., De Lange, N., & Moletsane, R. (2016). Me and my cellphone: Constructing change from the inside through cellphilms and participatory video in a rural community. *Area, 48*(4), 435–441. <https://doi.org/10.1111/area.12142>

Mitchell, C., De Lange, N., & Moletsane, R. (2017). *Participatory visual methodologies: Social change, community and policy.* SAGE. <https://doi.org/10.1080/17441692.2016.1170184>

Noble, A., Owens, B., Thulien, N., & Suleiman, A. (2022). "I feel like I'm in a revolving door, and COVID has made it spin a lot faster": The impact of the COVID-19 pandemic on youth experiencing homelessness in Toronto, Canada. *Plos one, 17*(8). Article e0273502. <https://doi.org/10.1371/journal.pone.0273502>

Nowicka-Sauer, K. (2007). Patients' perspective: Lupus in patients' drawings: Assessing drawing as a diagnostic and therapeutic method. *Clinical Rheumatology, 26*, 1523–1525.

Parks, C. D. (2020). Group dynamics when battling a pandemic. *Group Dynamics: Theory, Research, and Practice, 24*(3), 115.

Salmon, S., Taillieu, T. L., Fortier, J., Stewart-Tufescu, A., & Afifi, T. O. (2022). Pandemic-related experiences, mental health symptoms, substance use, and relationship conflict among older adolescents and young adults from Manitoba, Canada. *Psychiatry Research, 311*. Article 114495. <https://doi.org/10.1016/j.psychres.2022.114495>

Schön, D. A. (1983). *The reflective practitioner: How professionals think in action.* Basic Books.

Sheikhan, N. Y., Hawke, L. D., Ma, C., Courtney, D., Szatmari, P., Cleverley, K., Voineskos, A., Cheung, A., & Henderson, J. (2022). A longitudinal cohort study of youth mental health and substance use before and during the COVID-19 pandemic in Ontario, Canada: An exploratory analysis. *The Canadian Journal of Psychiatry, 67*(11), 842–854. Article 07067437221097906. <https://doi.org/10.1177/07067437221097906>

Singh, R., Rodrigues, A., Webb, C., & Grady, R. (2022). The impact of the COVID-19 pandemic on number and severity of new diagnoses of restrictive eating disorders during prolonged lockdown in Ontario, Canada. *Journal of Adolescent Health, 70*(4), S81-S82.

Stewart, S. L., Vasudeva, A. S., Van Dyke, J. N., & Poss, J. W. (2022). Child and youth mental health needs and service utilization during COVID-19. *Traumatology, 28*(3), 311–324.

Switzer, S. (2020). "People give and take a lot in order to participate in things:" Youth talk back–making a case for non-participation. *Curriculum Inquiry, 50*(2), 168–193.

Tuck, E. (2009). Suspending damage: A letter to communities. *Harvard Educational Review, 79*(3), 409–428.

Tuck, E., & Yang, K. W. (2014). Unbecoming claims: Pedagogies of refusal in qualitative research. *Qualitative Inquiry*, *20*(6), 811–818.

UNICEF Canada. (2020). *U-Report Canada: Impacts of the COVID-19 pandemic on young people in Canada—poll 1: How young people are experiencing the pandemic*. United Nations. <https://oneyouth.unicef.ca/sites/default/files/2020-05/U-Report_COVID-19_Poll_2_Results_external.pdf>

Vanner, C., Holloway, A., J. Mitchell C. & Altenberg, J. (2022). Round and round the carousel papers: Facilitating a visual interactive dialogue with young people. In C. Burkholder, J. Aledebi & J. Schwab-Cartas (Eds.). *Leading and listening to community: Facilitating qualitative, arts-based & visual research for social change*. Routledge.

Weaver, B., Thorpe, A., Mandrona, A., MacEntee, K., & Burkholder, C. (2022). Theorizing Non-Participation in a Mail-Based Participatory Visual Research Project with 2SLGBTQ+ Youth in Atlantic Canada. In C. Burkholder, J. Aledebi & J. Schwab-Cartas (Eds.). *Leading and listening to community: Facilitating qualitative, arts-based & visual research for social change* (pp. 127–141). Routledge.

Weinberg, H. (2020). Online group psychotherapy: Challenges and possibilities during COVID-19—A practice review. *Group Dynamics: Theory, Research, and Practice*, *24*(3), 201–211.

· 3 ·

"THEY'RE KIND OF LOSING IT": YOUNG PERFECTIONISTS' MENTAL HEALTH EXPERIENCES DURING THE FIRST COVID-19 LOCKDOWN

Dawn Zinga, Danielle S. Molnar,
Melissa Blackburn, and Natalie Tacuri

Perfectionism, Mental Health, and COVID-19

Adolescence and young adulthood are critical times during which individuals move from being primarily reliant on parents to seeking more autonomy and social relationships with others outside their family. School, social, recreational, and work environments provide avenues for young people to develop more autonomy, and they are key in supporting growth in self-regulation and social connection. Unfortunately, the COVID-19 pandemic disrupted these environments, impacting young peoples' growth and development as well as their access to friends, supports, and resources outside the home.

Unsurprisingly, many studies have identified a range of mental health impacts on youth during the pandemic. Some studies found improvements in mental health (Widnall et al., 2020) or a pattern of increases and decreases in mental health problems (Knowles et al., 2022; Raw et al., 2021). However, many studies reported increased symptoms of depression, anxiety, and/or loneliness (Branquinho et al., 2020; Ellis et al., 2020; Vaillancourt et al., 2022; Villanti et al., 2022; Wang et al., 2020). Further, although virtual peer interaction may be compensatory, concerns have also been raised that youth may have been disproportionately impacted by restricted face-to-face interactions (Orben et al., 2020). Indeed, research suggests that despite contact via technological means, youth experienced a social contact deficit during lockdowns (Larivière-Bastien et al., 2022).

Samji et al. (2022) recognized that while there were fluctuating patterns across countries, there was an overall trend toward declining mental health and that some youth were more at risk than others due to pre-existing conditions and specific contexts. Specifically, Samji et al. (2022) identified older adolescents, girls, and youth who experienced neurodiversity or chronic conditions as being more at risk for poorer mental health outcomes. Similarly, Raw et al. (2021) identified youth with special education needs or neurodevelopmental disorders as being particularly at risk during the pandemic. Knowles et al. (2022) further identified greater risk for youth living in challenging circumstances (e.g., experiencing financial struggles and/or poor housing situations), those directly affected by the pandemic, and those who expressed multiple areas of concern about pandemic conditions (e.g., having to stay home, not seeing friends, not having enough money, getting sick). Notably, young people with pre-existing mental health concerns (e.g., stress, anxiety, mood disorders, ADHD, autism) prior to the pandemic were also identified as being at higher risk for poorer mental health outcomes during the pandemic (Jefsen et al., 2020).

Collectively, research indicates that the pandemic had profound effects on young people. Yet, evidence supports heterogeneity in responses to the pandemic conditions among youth, underscoring the importance of taking individual differences into account. A key individual difference that may help account for this heterogeneity among young people is *perfectionism*, defined as the deeply engrained requirement of perfection from the self and/or others (Hewitt & Flett, 1991).

Perfectionism

Several conceptualizations and models of perfectionism abound among adults and youth (see Flett et al., 2022). However, researchers generally agree that perfectionism is a complex personality style that operates at the other-relational, self-relational, and dispositional levels (Hewitt et al., 2017; Molnar et al., 2023a). At the other-relational level, concentration is placed on perfectionistic behavior in the form of perfectionistic self-presentation, which reflects the propensity for some perfectionists to engage in active self-promotion of a perfect image while concealing any perceived flaws from others (Hewitt et al., 2003). In contrast, at the self-relational level, the focus is on the frequency in which people experience automatic perfectionistic thoughts centered on the need to be perfect, self-neglect and, in extreme cases, self-harm (Flett et al., 1998). Finally, at the dispositional level, perfectionism is conceptualized as operating as an enduring personality trait that has a pervasive impact on the self (Hewitt & Flett, 1991).

Arguably, researchers tend to show a strong bias toward conceptualizing perfectionism as a deeply entrenched multidimensional personality trait that influences all aspects of the self (i.e., dispositional level). Among youth, this is most commonly conceptualized as demanding perfection from the self or others (Flett et al., 2016) and can be thought of among adolescents as consisting of both intrapersonal and interpersonal elements (Flett et al., 2016; Molnar et al., 2023a). Self-oriented perfectionism (SOP) is intrapersonal and represents an internally driven need to be flawless, whereas socially prescribed perfectionism (SPP) is interpersonal and represents an individual's belief that perfectionism is required by significant others who will respond harshly if the perfectionistic standards are not met (Flett et al., 2016). As we have argued elsewhere (see Molnar et al., 2023a), the conceptualizations and measures of perfectionism have been largely derived from adult samples and dominated by quantitative approaches. In our qualitative research with young perfectionists, we mindfully opted to use self-definitions of perfectionism and not quantitative measures. Thus, participants identified as "perfectionists" according to their own understandings of what "perfectionist" means to them and were not provided with any of the conceptualizations offered within the perfectionism literature. Such an approach is not unprecedented (see Hill et al., 2015; Slaney & Ashby, 1996) and offers more insight into the experience of perfectionism by individuals. Consequently, we have not adopted a particular conceptualization of perfectionism in this chapter as our research focused on self-identified perfectionists.

Perfectionism and the Pandemic

Flett and Hewitt (2020) posited that individuals high in perfectionism would have a particularly difficult time adjusting to pandemic conditions because they are highly reactive to stress, do not respond well to uncertainty, and have limited self-regulation and coping skills. Recent research has confirmed that perfectionism placed adolescents and emerging adults at greater risk for psychological distress during the COVID-19 pandemic (Flett, 2021; Flett & Hewitt, 2020; Hill & Madigan, 2022; Levine et al., 2022; Molnar et al., 2021, 2023c). In some of our earlier work (Molnar et al., 2023c), we found that adolescents higher in SOP and SPP were more vulnerable to experiencing negative impacts from the pandemic, such as higher levels of anxiety and depressive symptoms and that stress was an explanatory pathway linking perfectionism to greater psychological distress. However, work examining perfectionism in youth in the context of the pandemic has thus far been predominantly quantitative (Hill & Madigan, 2022; Iancheva et al., 2020; Levine et al., 2022; Molnar et al., 2021, 2023c; see Blackburn et al., 2022, for an exception). Consequently, this chapter aims to fill this gap by employing qualitative inquiry to center the voices of young perfectionists in research focusing on their experiences during the early stages of the pandemic.

Methods

This chapter focuses on the positive and negative mental health outcomes associated with the COVID-19 pandemic conditions among adolescent self-identified perfectionists, along with the strategies that these youth discussed to manage their mental health during the pandemic. The work presented here is part of a larger, qualitative research project that aimed to examine how young perfectionists define, perceive, and experience perfectionism in their lives and more specifically during the pandemic.

Recruitment

Participants were recruited via online social media postings and through an online article featuring the study in the university newspaper. Youth were eligible for the study if they self-identified as a perfectionist and were between the ages of 13 and 25 years. Individuals' self-identification as perfectionists was based on their understanding of themselves and of perfectionism, an approach that has been used successfully by Hill et al. (2015) and Molnar et al. (2023a). This study received approval from the Brock University Research Ethics Board and all participants consented (18 years and above) or assented (17 years and younger with parental consent provided) to participate in the research before the interview was scheduled.

Participants

There were 58 young perfectionists who completed the study and whose data are included in our analyses. The sample was primarily female (n = 53; 91.4%) with the remaining participants identifying as male, and their ages ranged from 13 to 24 years (M = 17.04 SD = 2.84). The youth were predominantly white (n = 47; 81.1%), followed by Asian Canadians (n = 4; 6.9%), Latin Canadians (n = 1; 1.7%), Indigenous Peoples in Canada (n = 1; 1.7%), and others (n = 4; 6.9%). One participant did not report their race (1.7%).

For the analyses, we divided the participants into two groups reflecting their educational experiences. The first group, pre-postsecondary, consisted of 35 participants (2 men and 33 women) who were enrolled in upper elementary (7 participants in Grades 7–8) or secondary education (28 participants in Grades 9–12). The second group, postsecondary plus, included 23 participants (3 men and

20 women) who were either enrolled in postsecondary (n = 17), recent graduates (n = 2), or had completed postsecondary and were either working or laid-off due to the pandemic conditions (n = 4).

Procedure

Interviews were conducted in May and June 2020 during the first pandemic lockdown in Ontario, Canada. Each semi-structured interview was conducted online using Lifesize software and was audio and video recorded for transcription purposes. Interviews were facilitated by the first, third, and fourth authors and three graduate-level research assistants. Upon completion of the interview, participants were provided with a link to complete a short demographic survey, after which they were sent a $40 (CAD) gift card via email.

All participants completed a detailed two-part semi-structured interview that lasted between 90 and 120 minutes. After careful consideration, we opted not to ask youth directly about their mental health during the pandemic and instead focused on their pandemic experiences at home and in school as well as their approach to pandemic rules and procedures. One part of the interview focused on COVID-19 experiences and the other part focused on how participants conceptualized and experienced perfectionism.

The COVID-19 portion of the interview focused on participants' overall experiences during the first lockdown and included questions about lockdown protocols, school experiences, and impacts of the pandemic on their social lives. While none of the interview questions asked participants about their mental health during the pandemic, youth still chose to speak about mental health throughout the interview. The conversations about mental health comprise the data analyzed in this study. Names presented here are pseudonyms.

Data Analysis and Reflexivity

Following transcription, anonymized interview transcripts were uploaded to NVivo (QSR International Pty Ltd, 2020). During this process, the interviews were entered as two separate transcripts for each participant in recognition of the two distinct sections of the interview. The data analyzed in this chapter is drawn from the pandemic experiences section of the interview and not from the conceptualization and experience of perfectionism part of the interview. Consensus coding (Zinga et al., 2013) was combined with inductive thematic analysis (Braun & Clarke, 2006) to code and analyze the data. It is important to note that we undertook a social constructionist approach, as we focused on unpacking the realities expressed by the adolescents about their experiences (Braun & Clarke, 2021).

As we were particularly interested in how young perfectionists conceptualized and described their pandemic-related experiences, an inductive approach was most appropriate because it positions the analysis as being driven by the data and not by existing theoretical constructions such as the various theories of perfectionism. Similarly, we identify as taking a social constructionist approach because it captures how we focused on unpacking realities within the data. Given our focus on self-identification and not deductively placing theoretical conceptualization onto the data, these approaches were key to achieving our goal of understanding conceptualizations and experiences of perfectionism from the perspective of the young people who experience it daily. As such, our approach was informed by, but did not exclusively follow Braun and Clarke's (2006; 2021) approach to reflexive thematic analysis.

Our analysis followed the six phases (i.e., becoming familiar with the data, coding, initial theme creation, development/review of themes, refining/finalizing themes, writing up) identified by Braun and Clarke (2021). Our process began with each analysis team member reviewing several transcripts to identify potential emergent codes (i.e., familiarizing). In a series of brainstorming meetings, the potential emergent codes were shared and discussed until consensus was reached surrounding codes and a coding guide was developed (i.e., coding). Discussions and brainstorming continued throughout the subsequent coding process during which we maintained an audit trail that distinguished between direct responses to questions and emergent material. Our discussion then turned to a focus on patterns and themes in the data (i.e., initial theme creation) and continued as we further developed and reviewed themes until we reached a consensus on our revised themes and moved to capture the analysis in writing.

In the following section, we present the results from our analysis, which were organized into themes related to positive mental health, negative mental health, and strategies that perfectionistic youth discussed as associated with COVID-19 pandemic conditions. Results about health-promoting behaviors among perfectionistic youth during the COVID-19 pandemic (Blackburn et al., 2022) and conceptualizations of perfectionism (Molnar et al., 2023a) are reported elsewhere.

Results

We identified mental health as a dominant theme in participants' pandemic experiences interviews, and we organized the data on mental health into seven sub-themes: change in pace; focus on the self; isolation, social disconnection, and negative emotion; stress and anxiety; lack of motivation; awareness of others struggling; and strategies. Additionally, our results include a group-based analysis that considered the similarities and differences in how individuals from the two groups (i.e., pre-postsecondary and postsecondary plus) discussed mental health across the seven sub-themes.

Change in Pace

Interestingly, participants identified the break associated with pandemic lockdown as having positive impacts on their mental health. Four postsecondary plus participants described how the break from demanding schedules resulted in stress reduction while providing an opportunity to reflect on and adjust behaviors and schedules. As Soraya (age 20) indicated, "I'm staying healthy and happy, and well," while Lyli (24) spoke to self-reflection saying, "that's been very positive because I think I'm establishing routines that are healthy and that I can carry beyond the pandemic." Mary (20) described how "I've learned how to control my stress and my urges to push myself ... because I had the time to relax and take a break." Susan (19) attributed her positive mental health to the lockdown, "my mental health is 100%," as being one of the benefits of having extra time at home during the pandemic.

This break from routine and associated stress relief was echoed by nine pre-postsecondary girls. Emma (14) spoke about having more free time and stated, "I've been able to relax more and it's really helped my mental health" while Brenna (16) reported, "I have been significantly less stressed ... my life isn't as chaotic as it normally is." Both indicated that the pandemic restrictions interrupted their usual routines, resulting in a forced break that suspended some stress and pressure.

Unlike the postsecondary plus group who spoke in more general terms, several pre-postsecondary girls identified specific pressures relieved by the pandemic conditions. Aria (15) enjoyed not worrying about others' opinions: "I don't have to worry about what other people are going to think of me ... I'm not trying to impress people from home." Dana (15) also spoke to being relieved of some school pressure: "it's harder for me when I'm in person to hand in an assignment ... now I'm not as concerned about that. I'm kind of just 'yeah, that's my work. It's good enough.'"

In addition, many of the pre-postsecondary participants spoke about the positive impact being limited to the beginning of the restrictions. For example, Amy (13) said, "it's been joy at the beginning." Bella (14) seemed to agree: "for like the first like two months... it was delightful." Similarly, Ava (15) said, "at first, I was really happy about [not attending school] ... but now that we've been without it for a long time, I miss it." All of them indicated that the positive mental health effects faded away as the restrictions continued, which is when they became associated with stress and other negative mental health impacts.

Focus on the Self

Distinct from the reflection on routines and behaviors described above, participants also spoke about positive mental health impacts associated with time to
focus on themselves, which seemed to have had a longer lasting impact. Twelve
participants, including eight postsecondary plus and four pre-postsecondary,
discussed working on themselves and getting to know themselves better. Lyli (24)
said, "it's given me a lot of time to reflect on my own personal development," and
Bella (14) explained that "[I] just get a deeper understanding of myself." Similarly,
Aria (15) said, "I really got to work on myself."

Lyli (24), one of the participants in postsecondary plus, described guilt around
self-focus being lessened during lockdown, saying "it's given me the chance and
the space and the time to not feel guilty about working on myself." This sense of
productively using time to focus on the self was commonly cited by participants
in both groups. For example, Julie (20) said, "well, since I've had like all this time
to myself and that I'm not normally used to, I definitely focus more on myself."
Similarly, Charlotte (17) explained, "I'm reflecting most on what I need to be
happy and healthy because I didn't have the time to look at that before because of
how busy I was." Interestingly, one person from each group spoke of self-image in
connection to self-focus during the pandemic. Terri (18) valued the opportunity
to work on herself without "external opinions and stuff" intruding, and Aria (15)
spoke of valuing the opportunity to develop "a better self-image of myself." Both
referenced the isolation and space from others offered by the pandemic as beneficial for working on the self without the degree of external input they experienced
during their regular routines.

Isolation, Social Disconnection, and Negative Emotion

Participants in both groups identified isolation and social disconnection as having
negative impacts on their mental health and, more specifically, through increased
negative emotions. All postsecondary plus individuals and 12 from the younger
group referred to sadness and depression or directly identified mental health challenges associated with the lockdown conditions. This included comments such as:
"I get lonely, I get sad … it's a never-ending spiral" (Stella, 18); "it has been hard
mentally… at nights I cry in my bed" (Anna, 13); "I knew that I was really upset.
So I went on a drive and I parked my car and I cried" (Gaby, 18).

The connection between negative mental health and social isolation was
explicitly discussed by six of the postsecondary plus participants and seven of
the pre-postsecondary participants. Stacey (19) spoke about finally connecting
to her peers in her university residence only to have to leave, "so when we finally

connected ... it got shut down and everyone went their separate ways. So it was sad, getting disconnected." Sean (20) talked about the struggle of being disconnected: "I'm very outgoing ... so it's been the hardest, the hardest days of my life." Mary (20) and Chloe (16) both spoke of feeling lonely and disconnected. This was shared by Ellie (17), Faith (17), and Callie (17) who all spoke of feeling forcibly withdrawn from their preferred social interaction patterns and feeling as if they had gone from vibrant social lives to nothing.

In contrast, three individuals, two from postsecondary plus and one from pre-postsecondary, talked about responding to pandemic conditions by actively withdrawing and engaging in social isolation. Brenna (16) spoke of withdrawing from others: "I have cut myself off a little bit from talking to people." This was even more prominent for Terri (18) who said, "I'd say keeping away like just isolating, even from my family. I just wanted, being alone and not talking to people." Stella (18) said, "so then I tell myself, well I'm sad so I don't want to see anyone or talk to anyone."

With respect to loss, three participants, two from postsecondary plus and one pre-postsecondary, specifically identified pandemic-associated losses. Gabby (18) was in her senior year in high school and spoke of missed milestones: "I'm more upset about like the experiences that I have been looking forward to since forever ... that's the most challenging part. Being sad and angry... that I'm missing the things that everyone else is going to get." Sean (20) also spoke about specific losses tied to his growth into adulthood: "I just got this job. I just got this apartment. I lost basically all my passions and everything that I love doing. No sports, no income. I lost it all." Hilary (18) was also grieving lost experiences, as she was in first year of her university and enjoying dorm life when classes were canceled: "I have never cried more in my life than that whole thing. I remember I woke up and then, the day before, [my university] had canceled their classes then my school canceled."

One specific loss identified by both groups was the loss of human touch or comfort. Lacey (18) spoke about wanting to comfort her friends during the pandemic: "I feel like I want to give them a hug, but I can't." Similarly, both Sean (20) and Ellie (17) missed hugging friends as part of regular socializing, wishing that they could give them a hug. However, Soraya (20) spoke to a more complex sense of loss around human contact:

> It's like everybody's afraid of each other right now, it seems like, and I feel like it just makes you feel so uncomfortable. [...] I definitely am looking forward to just hugging everybody again and not being afraid of other people.

Soraya's comments speak to not only the loss of physical contact, but the fear of being close to other people. Fears linked to pandemic conditions and the associated stress and anxiety were so common that they formed their own sub-theme.

Stress and Anxiety

Talking about stress and anxiety was more common in the pre-postsecondary group, as nine young women and two young men spoke about anxiety, whereas only five postsecondary plus women spoke of stress or anxiety. However, participants in both groups spoke of stress and anxiety associated with fears of things not returning to normal and of the future more generally. Julie (20) was stressed by pandemic conditions and wanted her "normal life" back, while Nicole (24) spoke of "the fear that maybe life will always be this way." Those in the younger group like Ellie (17) also expressed fear of the future: "I would say feeling very stressed out about the future." Some future-oriented fears were more specific, as exemplified by Emma (14) who was anxious about the uncertainty in her life around schooling and the pandemic more generally, "just fear of not knowing what's going to happen for this pandemic … but we're not quite sure if it's going to be extended or if we're going to continue with schooling." Amy (13), who was finishing grade eight, worried about her future in high school and her current lack of socializing: "my social anxiety gets really, really bad and I just can't function well. And that's not going to be good for a high school with 900 kids who, most of them, I haven't met."

School-oriented stress and anxiety were prevalent in both groups, with online schooling being the main concern. In the postsecondary plus group, Layla (20) reported being stressed and not enjoying her online experiences: "I'm doing online courses right now and I don't like it. So it makes me stressed out for this semester." Soraya (20) was worried about her upcoming semester: "fall term is going to be mainly online. That gives me so much anxiety." Lucy (18) was stressed about how her existing anxieties could handle the added stress of being online, saying that "I have test anxiety and essay anxiety … I've worked with therapists; I've worked with people at school about it. But I don't know how to fix it."

As noted above, stress was particularly pronounced within the pre-postsecondary group, and participants described various ways in which stress manifested and impacted their daily lives. Avery (16) talked about being overwhelmed: "they post everything all at once, it's really overwhelming." Similarly, Amy (13) spoke of chaos: "then they started doing online schooling and that's when everything went to chaos. That's where my anxiety started acting out, my perfectionism got worse." Ellie (17) worried about her progress, saying: "I feel stressed out. I feel like I'm falling behind and I'm not retaining as well as I normally do." Colton (16) agreed with stress associated with understanding as he said, "I feel online school can sometimes be a little more stressful because there's some mystery to it that you're not 100% understanding it." Chloe (16) captured multiple stresses associated with schooling and the pandemic:

When I didn't have any work, I was a mess. It was not pretty. I was freaking out. It was not great. I was worried about my schoolwork … Just things were weird, and nothing was normal. It [online schooling] gives me a lot of time to just be even more stressed out about everything and my grades and stuff. And it's giving me a lot more time to just do the same thing over and over and over again. And it, I don't know, I can't really stop myself from not doing that anymore.

Like Chloe (16), Anna (13) talked about the stress of online school and the fear of falling behind. She also spoke to how her social isolation compounded these stresses, saying that "I'm an only child too … so it has been hard mentally … at nights I cry in my bed because it's so hard."

Pandemic behaviors and conditions were another source of stress and anxiety that was recounted by participants in this study. However, these accounts were predominantly from the pre-postsecondary group, with only Julie (20) and Soraya (20) from the postsecondary plus group voicing anxiety about current conditions. Soraya spoke of trying to control her anxiety about the pandemic when she talked about "not worrying about how stressed out and depressed I am over the situation." In contrast, Julie (20) discussed more specific sources of anxiety, "like some businesses are allowing to be opened back up again and they don't have good health protocols of dealing with the virus, which makes me nervous."

In contrast, many individuals in the pre-postsecondary group associated stress and anxiety with pandemic behaviors and conditions. Ben (17) spoke about his anxiety and frustration around friends ignoring the pandemic restrictions and continuing to socialize, which "stressed me and frustrated me a lot because I was doing what they [government] asked and they were not." Aria (15) reported getting overwhelmed by shopping trips and stressed by her mother's meandering approach, saying "that kind of overwhelms me because I just wanted to get in and kind of get out." Aria also worried about being exposed to a lot of people and people getting too close in the store. Fiona (14) was stressed by how people walked in groups, explaining that "there's too many people and it stresses me out a lot … I feel bad that I can't help fix it, other than stay at home." Fiona (14) was overwhelmed by news about current conditions: "I don't like to watch too much of it or it becomes very stressful for me."

Lack of Motivation

Several participants discussed feeling a lack of motivation during the pandemic, though only one individual from the postsecondary plus group talked about this. Sean (20) said he was "just feeling useless and not getting anything done. So, it's sometimes hard to be motivated to get things done … like I could go on a run, but I'm not really motivated to do it."

All other mentions of amotivation occurred in the pre-postsecondary group, where it was reported by six participants. Claire (18) connected her lack of routine with being unproductive: "I think just because there's no routine right now, it kind of makes you feel unproductive and the motivation to do schoolwork is definitely very low right now." Grace (16) spoke of struggling with motivation to do schoolwork, saying, "I haven't been doing all my work because I don't feel motivated." In both cases, there was a link between motivation and the ability to be productive.

In contrast, Amanda (15) and Avery (16) discussed a lack of motivation but associated it with spending more time in bed or being tired. Amanda reported, "I'm in my bed more, it's really sad. I wish I was motivated to go out and do something," and Avery said, "I've been more tired lately. So I've been waking up very, very late ... then I don't feel motivated to work at all." Brenna (16) offered a slightly different perspective as she spoke of heightened procrastination and active avoidance: "I guess motivationally, I don't want to do my schoolwork ... and I've noticed my procrastination has increased severely ... I'm not talking to any of my friends either." Ellie (17) stood out as experiencing anhedonia rather than just lack of motivation. Specifically, she spoke about her inability to enjoy activities that she normally enjoyed doing:

> A lot of the things that I feel passionate about, I don't really feel passionate about at the moment. I like to write as well and I literally cannot do it. Like I cannot sit at the piano and play or I cannot write a poem ... I'm having a really, really hard time doing the things that I know I enjoy. But right now, I don't even feel like I enjoy them.

Awareness of Others Struggling

Participants in both groups were aware of how others were struggling, although this was more pronounced in the postsecondary plus group (with eight individuals) than in the pre-postsecondary group (with two individuals). Both Colton (16) and Charlotte (17) explicitly indicated an awareness of others' struggles with pandemic conditions stating, "I can definitely see with other people that they're kind of losing it" and "I know people have struggled with it, especially kids my age," respectively. Some of the postsecondary plus group also had more general comments such as "I'm not struggling as much as other people are" (Tanya, 20), "it was bad because people's mental health stuff was affected" (Stacey, 19), and "I know a lot of other people are struggling" (Susan, 19).

However, the postsecondary plus group tended to offer more nuanced and specific observations about others' struggles. Some, like Lucy (18), disagreed with isolation measures: "I don't agree with social distancing, just because I know so many people have been struggling because of this." Others discussed ways to reach out and connect remotely. Rachel (19) spoke of how she supports others who are struggling by "text[ing] them here and there, just saying, how's it going and see how they're doing and handling it." Some specifically mentioned the benefits of posting online. Soraya (20) said, "it does help to see other kids my age talking about, whether it be on Twitter or on Instagram, just talking about how they've been struggling a lot with their mental health," and Susan (19) spoke of posting "these videos on my Instagram to help other people about mental illness and stuff." Lacey (18) recognized the struggles of her younger friends who were missing milestones and felt bad about not being able to physically be there for them, saying, "that's hard cause sometimes the only thing that makes people feel better is just your presence and that's not really possible." Lacey who was also worried about a particular friend who was not coping well, made an important point: "nobody really knows how everyone's dealing with things." She also recognized her own resistance to accepting pandemic realities: "I should have been more empathetic of how you guys were all feeling super sad … it took me a while to accept that this was actually happening."

Strategies

Participants' awareness of struggles associated with the pandemic prompted a discussion about the strategies that young people were using to cope. Sixteen individuals, nine postsecondary plus and seven pre-postsecondary, spoke about what they were doing to cope with pandemic conditions and associated challenges. The common thread across the two groups was the use of self-care activities. Many referenced physical activities such as working out, including Tanya (20) who said, "I get in at least five workouts a week, just to help me mentally and physically." Participants also talked about other physical activities such as walking, yoga, or sports. Ava (15) said she would reach out to others as a coping strategy, as did Soraya (20) and Chloe (16). For example, Soraya (20) spoke about "maintaining [her] therapy" as well as reaching out virtually through social media to engage with others, and Chloe (16) said she connected with trusted others: "[I] talk with my parents if I'm getting really freaked out about everything." Emma (14) and Diane (16) from the pre-postsecondary group spoke about strategies such as deep breathing and journaling.

Two participants discussed the importance of keeping busy, and three others focused on schedules. Chloe (16) said it was important to have at least one thing she could do if she felt bored, while Rose (18) stressed the importance of staying busy: "I think the most beneficial thing is just keeping busy right now. Or else I'll just feel more wrapped up in my own head." Lucy (18), Lacey (18), and Callie (17) emphasized needing a schedule to stay on track. Lucy (18) said, "the night before, I set out like a timed schedule, it's kind of part of my OCD," whereas Lacey (18) stressed that having a work schedule kept her grounded. Callie (17) also focused on the importance of schedules: "I like to plan my day before it starts. Or else I get kind of like anxious."

In contrast, several individuals spoke to a less structured approach, such as Fiona (14), who used fun to keep her distracted and enhance her mental balance: "[I] try to do fun things that keep me entertained, just make me feel sort of stable." Avery (16) and Mary (20) also took a less structured approach and focused on taking breaks and relaxing. Regardless of the type of strategy used, most participants actively tried to manage the negative impacts of the pandemic and work toward maintaining or achieving positive mental health.

Discussion

In line with theoretical assertions (see Flett & Hewitt, 2020), a growing body of work is beginning to show that young people higher in perfectionism are experiencing greater psychological distress during the COVID-19 pandemic compared to their less perfectionistic peers (Flett, 2021; Flett & Hewitt, 2020; Hill & Madigan, 2022; Levine et al., 2022; Molnar et al., 2021, 2023c). This extends pre-pandemic research that has established perfectionism as a vulnerability factor for poorer mental health (Limburg et al., 2017). Moreover, empirical evidence supports the Perfectionism Diathesis-Stress Model (Flett et al., 1995), which postulates that perfectionism is particularly aversive under high levels of stress (Flett & Hewitt, 2020). However, we currently lack an in-depth understanding of how and why young perfectionists have experienced particularly high levels of psychopathology during the pandemic. Thus, the primary aim of this chapter is to use qualitative methodology to draw attention to the voices of young perfectionists to better understand their experiences during the COVID-19 pandemic.

Although mental health was not directly addressed during our in-depth interviews with self-identified young perfectionists, our participants offered a rich and nuanced discussion of their mental health experiences during the first pandemic lockdown. These young perfectionists did express some improvements in mental health during the early stages of the pandemic in the form of stress reduction due to getting a break from their typically busy schedules and time to engage in self-reflection; however, these benefits tended to largely dissipate over time as the pandemic progressed. Moreover, the mental health problems discussed by participants, including experiencing a lack of motivation along with high levels of negative emotion, stress, and anxiety, appeared to be more prevalent and more enduring compared to any mental health gains.

Perfectionists' Nuanced Accounts of Their Mental Health During the COVID-19 Pandemic

While we believe that the seven sub-themes of mental health identified in this work are representative of the young self-identified perfectionists who participated in this study, it is important to highlight the high degree of heterogeneity in young perfectionists' experiences during the early phases of the pandemic. For example, many self-identified perfectionists spoke of the benefits offered by the change of pace that resulted from the government-mandated lockdowns. However, some key points of divergence emerged such that some participants, such as Mary (20) and Bella (14), spoke of the change of pace offering them stress relief because they had fewer obligations and more time to focus on themselves. However, other participants who appeared to be overly concerned with others discovering any of their potential flaws specifically identified experiencing respite from the in-person pressures they experienced from worrying about other people's opinions. This propensity was expressed by Terri (18) and Aria (15), who both expressed relief because social isolation limited their exposure to other people's opinions and meant that they did not have to worry about how they were presenting themselves. Furthermore, while many participants spoke of pandemic conditions as isolating and interfering with social connection and expressed a strong desire to be with others, a few participants responded to the social isolation triggered by pandemic conditions with the tendency to actively withdraw even further than conditions required.

Although speculative at this point, these differences may be explained by how individuals experience their perfectionism, given that both theory and research support that young people tend to experience and manifest their perfectionism in unique and varied ways (Flett & Hewitt, 2022; Molnar et al., 2023a). For instance, Levine et al. (2022) pointed to heterogeneity in experiences among young perfectionists wherein individuals higher in self-critical perfectionism (akin to SPP) experienced increased depressive symptoms and individuals higher in personal standards perfectionism (akin to SOP) experienced reduced depressive standards, felt more socially connected, competent, autonomous, and were better able to engage in new opportunities.

Similarly, Hill and Madigan (2022) found differences in how adolescent perfectionists experienced the pandemic. Their study revealed that negative reactions to imperfection (an indicator of perfectionistic concerns, which is akin to SPP) and anti-mattering were associated with higher stress and poorer self-regulation of at-home learning, whereas perfectionistic strivings (akin to SOP) were related to better self-regulation. This was also reflected in our participants as there was a tendency for some participants to discuss their perfectionism as being beneficial to their self-regulation, especially when their perfectionism was directed at being more productive. This was particularly notable among individuals who channeled their perfectionistic ways into self-improvement, such as Terri (18), Aria (15), and Lyli (24). Mary (20) also exemplified this as she described how her focus on self-improvement meant that "I haven't stressed myself out beyond repair … I've learned how to control my stress and my urges to push myself." This was linked to positive mental health impacts, as both pre-postsecondary and postsecondary plus youth indicated that the first lockdown provided time and space to focus more on the self, which resulted in some positive impacts such as better self-regulation, stress reduction, and self-improvement.

Both pre-postsecondary and postsecondary plus participants identified improvements in mental health that they associated with a break from their routines and associated stresses. However, the postsecondary plus group discussed these in a more generalized way, whereas the pre-postsecondary group tended to be more specific and conceptualized these gains as having a time-limited nature that was dissipating before the lockdown conditions were lifted. Again, heterogeneity in the experiences of young perfectionists was evident as Chloe (16) reported a decrease in mental health when her routine was disrupted: "when I didn't have any work, I was a mess. It was not pretty. I was freaking out."

The Need to be Perfectly Productive During Lockdown

There was a clear sense that the time alone provided by the lockdown became increasingly connected to the need to use it wisely and productively as the lockdown persisted. Two individuals, Terri (18) and Aria (15), made specific connections to the pressures associated with SPP and the need to present oneself perfectly to others. They spoke of how their social isolation provided a break from other peoples' opinions and allowed them to enjoy self-reflection and work on themselves. This points to the likelihood that some perfectionists who strive to project a perfect image to others (e.g., those who are high in perfectionistic self-presentation) do not gain mental health benefits from their typical self-reflection and self-improvement efforts. Rather, their usual tendencies toward self-reflection and efforts at self-improvement are grounded in the perceived unrealistic standards of a generalized other that become yet another vehicle to display their perfectionism to others at the detriment of their self-concept and mental health.

It is important to note that among both pre-postsecondary and postsecondary plus participants, discussions of inner work framed the activities associated with self-reflection and self-improvement as being productive. This suggests that for perfectionists, self-focus during typical routines (e.g., when their schedules are not disrupted by the pandemic) may seem indulgent and be associated with guilt for not engaging in more productive tasks. However, self-focus was characterized as a productive task in the context of the first pandemic-related lockdown, filling otherwise idle time. This finding is consistent with the notion that perfectionists tend to feel high levels of pressure and immense responsibility to be exceptionally productive at all times and discount external circumstances (such as a global pandemic) that may limit their productivity (Flett & Hewitt, 2020). Indeed, the overwhelming need to be productive seen here was likely a coping mechanism that young perfectionists used to gain a sense of control under unpredictable and unprecedented circumstances.

"It's Been the Hardest, Hardest Days of my Life": Lockdown-Related Tolls on Perfectionists' Mental Health

The negative impacts of the lockdown were identified by perfectionistic youth as isolation, social disconnection, negative emotion, stress, anxiety, and lack of motivation. Both pre-postsecondary and postsecondary plus participants spoke of isolation, social disconnection, and negative emotions, with the experience of negative emotion being the most common shared element across the two groups.

In terms of social disconnection, while the perfectionistic youth spoke of connecting virtually with friends and using social media to reach out to others, they still experienced profound isolation and social disconnection. In addition to missing social interactions, participants also spoke of missing physical touch and physical closeness in their friendships. This is consistent with the broader literature, which shows that isolation, social disconnection, and missing the physical aspects of friendship were common experiences for young people during the pandemic (e.g., Larivière-Bastien et al., 2022). While social disconnection and loneliness have been reported as adverse consequences of pandemic conditions for youth in general, isolation due to government-mandated lockdowns implemented to help mitigate the spread of COVID-19 seemed to be particularly detrimental for perfectionistic youth in our study. This is consistent with the Perfectionism Social Disconnection Model (PSDM; Hewitt et al., 2006), which describes perfectionists as tending to feel socially isolated from others and this sense of social disconnection may be objective as a result of their hostile interpersonal style or subjective due to their particularly high levels of interpersonal sensitivity (Hewitt et al., 2006, 2017). Further, this conclusion is in line with Flett and

Hewitt's (2020) contention that perfectionists, who already struggle to connect with significant others, "may find it exceptionally difficult to cope with loneliness and separation anxiety as they are not more isolated than ever before" (p. 88) in the context of the COVID-19 pandemic. While our study did not include non-perfectionistic youth and therefore cannot make direct comparisons, it is likely that perfectionists were particularly vulnerable to feeling disconnected from others during the pandemic because the lockdowns and socially distancing measures put in place to lessen the spread of COVID-19 intensified their already entrenched sense of social disconnection (Flett & Hewitt, 2020).

A central tenet of the PSDM is that social disconnection experienced by perfectionists fuels the development of psychological distress (Hewitt et al., 2006; 2017). Empirical evidence supports this premise in both adults (e.g., Smith et al., 2020) and youth (Goya Arce & Polo, 2017; Magson et al., 2019; Roxborough et al., 2012). In line with this body of work, the experience of stress and anxiety was prominent in both pre-postsecondary and postsecondary plus youth and centered on fear of the unknown, school concerns, the online school context, and pandemic restrictions and conditions. The pre-postsecondary group appeared to have more pronounced stress and anxiety than the postsecondary plus group, suggesting that the older perfectionists may have more coping mechanisms or other elements in their lives that ameliorate their stress and anxiety. It is also possible that this difference was reflective of their perfectionistic identities and perceived level of control. In Molnar et al. (2023a), we found that adolescent perfectionists experienced more negative emotions when they perceived a lack of control. While the postsecondary plus group may have had more strategies because they are older and have more experience dealing with difficult situations, they also tended to have more control over their living situations and environments than the pre-postsecondary group. While more of the postsecondary plus individuals referred to sadness, depression, or mental health challenges, both groups discussed these concerns at length.

Motivational Deficits Among Perfectionists During Lockdown

Lack of motivation, which is a common feature of depression (Fervaha et al., 2016), also emerged as a notable mental health theme among young perfectionists during the early stages of the pandemic. Interestingly, lack of motivation was only reported by one postsecondary plus individual, whereas six pre-postsecondary individuals reported lack of motivation and awareness of motivational challenges as well as tendencies to actively avoid doing things or connecting with others. This finding may seem counterintuitive at first, as some forms of perfectionism, such as SOP, are often linked with higher levels of motivation among young people (Einstein et al., 2000; Stoeber & Rambow, 2007). Indeed, striving to reach excessively high standards is an important feature of perfectionism itself. Yet, it is vital to keep in mind that other forms of perfectionism, especially those that are externally driven (i.e., SPP), tend to be associated with amotivation (Appleton & Hill, 2012; Chang et al., 2016), given that socially prescribed perfectionists typically experience feelings of helplessness due to their beliefs that exceptionally high standards are being imposed on them by others and are therefore outside of their control.

Indeed, feeling a lack of control was particularly prevalent among young people during the early stages of the pandemic, as they experienced exceptionally high levels of uncertainty due to the unprecedented nature of the pandemic along with significant disruptions to their typical school and extra-curricular activities. Given that young perfectionists report that they have a strong need for control and order and that they often rely on the structure of the school day and use schedules to impose order and control in their lives to aid their perfectionistic strivings (Molnar et al., 2023a), it is understandable that some young perfectionists had their motivation undermined by the government-mandated lockdowns and other pandemic-related events. For example, the withdrawal of the structure of the school day, the uncertainty of the pandemic, and the hastily implemented online schooling all contributed to what Amy (13) described as "chaos." Thus, it is not surprising that some of our participants reported a lack of motivation along with increased stress and anxiety associated with conditions that they had no control over (e.g., school concerns, online schooling, pandemic conditions, restrictions) and fear of the unknown.

Age-Related Differences in Mental Health Awareness and Coping

There were a few other notable differences between pre-postsecondary and post-secondary plus youth. While not captured in the specific sub-themes, across the data, some of those in the older group relative to the younger group displayed a deeper knowledge of mental health and mental health advocacy, which was also reflected by a greater awareness of others struggling. This emerged as more of a flavor within the data than a robust sub-theme, pointing once again to heterogeneity as not all members of the older group shared the deeper knowledge and engagement in mental health advocacy. Those who did display this deeper knowledge and sense of advocacy were focused on their own mental health and support of others. They also tended to identify mental health strategies such as reaching out to specifically support others and social media support (e.g., Instagram videos) that differed from the dominant strategies most of the young people identified (e.g., self-care, physical activities, social interaction). Many of the strategies identified by both groups such as physical activities and spending time with others were also identified in other studies (Ellis et al., 2020; Larivière-Bastien et al., 2022; Samji et al., 2022). These strategies can inform future health interventions and support resources offered to young people, including self-identified perfectionists, in times of crisis.

Conclusions and Recommendations

To our knowledge, this is the first qualitative study to examine the mental health experiences of young self-identified perfectionists in the context of the COVID-19 pandemic. As such, it offers insight into how these young people conceptualized and perceived their experiences during pandemic conditions without imposing preconceived theoretical understandings of perfectionism. Our participants described experiencing some gains in mental health, but these seemed to be time-limited and specific to the very early stages of the pandemic. Young perfectionists also discussed experiencing vast declines in mental health that seemed to be driven in part by heightened levels of social disconnection, supporting the PSDM (Hewitt et al., 2006, 2017), and extending previous quantitative work in pre-pandemic conditions (e.g., Goya Arce & Polo, 2017; Magson et al., 2019; Roxborough et al., 2012). Previous research (Flett, 2021; Flett & Hewitt, 2020; Hill & Madigan, 2022; Levine et al., 2022; Molnar et al., 2021; Molnar et al., 2023c) has identified young perfectionists as having been at greater risk for negative outcomes during the pandemic compared to their non-perfectionistic peers. Our in-depth examination of the experiences of these young perfectionists offers insight into *how* and *why* other studies may have found young perfectionists to be at higher risk during this time.

With respect to supporting young perfectionists, both in the context of the pandemic and beyond, awareness of the negative outcomes and struggles associated with perfectionism among youth is a key first step. Despite well-established mental health challenges related to perfectionism (e.g., Limburg et al., 2017; Smith et al., 2021), society still tends to view perfectionism as a largely positive trait and encourages young people to strive toward it. One example of this is the cliché of using perfectionism as a person's key flaw in a job interview when in fact, between the lines, they are promoting it as a positive attribute. While research is still teasing apart the complexity around this positive bias toward characterizing perfectionism as a preferred trait, preliminary evidence suggests that while the adults around perfectionistic youth such as teachers and parents are aware of the negative impacts of perfectionism, they are also biased toward seeing it positively based on a conflation with academic performance and drive (e.g., Molnar et al., 2023b). Parents, teachers, and coaches can also inadvertently reinforce perfectionism and place increased pressure on perfectionistic youth by consistently calling attention to how they exceed expectations. This results in youth continuing to value perfectionism while invisibly struggling under the weight of trying to meet increasingly unrealistic expectations. This is particularly problematic given that perfectionistic individuals tend to tie their sense of self-worth with their accomplishments (e.g., Burns, 1980; Molnar et al., 2023a; Rozental, 2020; Shafran et al., 2016). Indeed, Flett and Hewitt (2022) note that, for perfectionistic youth, high standards for performance are not simply about getting a perfect grade or executing a skill perfectly, but rather that these goals are proxies for perfecting the self. Thus, when perfectionists are unable to reach these standards, they view it as a reflection of a failure of the self as a person. In other words, perfectionistic youth demonstrate a tendency to gauge their worth as a person based on their performance and accomplishments.

In the current work, this became particularly salient in the accounts of the youth participants when the context of the pandemic inhibited their ability to pursue their usual standards for performance. In some cases, this appeared to encourage some of the youth to engage in further exploration of their identities more holistically outside of their typical schedules and obligations. However, for others, the disruptions brought on by the pandemic were a source of negative emotions such as stress, anxiety, depression, and amotivation, when they were unable or unsure how to navigate this new landscape in a way that was compatible with their typical goals. This is in line with the predictions of Flett and Hewitt (2020), who theorized that young perfectionists would react to the pandemic in one of two ways. First, they posited that the uncertainty of the circumstances of the pandemic would amplify perfectionism among perfectionistic individuals in a futile attempt to regain control, in turn exacerbating the mental health and motivational difficulties they may have been experiencing pre-pandemic. However, they also noted that, for some individuals, the pandemic may "serve as a catalyst for positive change and actually abandoning perfectionism because they have grown closer to other people or perhaps have simply come to realize the folly of striving for absolute perfection rather than excellence" (p. 15). Although it is important to keep in mind that the pandemic did seem to negatively affect many perfectionistic youth's mental health, it is promising that some perfectionists were able to use this time as a period of reflection and acknowledge that they are persons of worth beyond their ability to achieve.

While we have indicated that self-reflection seemed to be a beneficial tool for young perfectionists in developing a more adaptive mindset and consequently developing a more positive and holistic view of the self during a stressful and unprecedented time, the scaffolding and other associated support of these strategies may be challenging to implement. Indeed, direct intervention with young perfectionists can be quite difficult. On the one hand, research and theory suggest that, in the long term, the best course of action to address perfectionism and its maladaptive correlates through direct therapeutic intervention that aims to both reduce perfectionism and address the mental health difficulties perfectionists are experiencing (e.g., Hewitt et al., 2015, 2017; Tasca et al., 2007). There are a variety of avenues for achieving these goals with young people within a therapeutic context, including lowering the importance of being perfect by highlighting the costs and dangers of perfectionism, fostering a growth mindset in which failures are reframed as opportunities for learning that are to be expected rather than deficits of the self, and promoting self-compassion as a method for countering harsh self-criticism (Flett & Hewitt, 2014).

However, despite the fact that many young perfectionists could benefit from therapeutic intervention, young perfectionists may also be unwilling to seek help due to the perception of admitting to struggling and requiring support as a flaw in and of itself (e.g., Dang et al., 2019; DeRosa, 2000; Flett & Hewitt, 2013, 2014; Hewitt et al., 2008). As such, although individual treatment would be best, one way to circumvent this aversion to help-seeking is through the implementation of universal, school-based programs that take a positive psychology approach to promoting resilience among youth more broadly rather than targeting perfectionistic youth specifically. When strategies such as fostering a growth mindset, focusing on process not product, managing expectations, and promoting self-care are structured into the educational environment and applied to all students, young perfectionists will be more likely to take them up. An added benefit of this approach is that it addresses other barriers to direct intervention experienced by many youth such as accessibility, financial costs, and societal or cultural stigma associated with individual therapeutic interventions.

It is worth noting that when young perfectionists do present for individual treatment with mental health professionals, the practitioner should be particularly mindful in acknowledging and addressing the defensive interpersonal style of perfectionistic clients to help establish a positive and safe therapeutic relationship with the young person (Hewitt et al., 2008, 2017). Additionally, it is important to keep in mind that, although there are common experiences among perfectionistic youth, there is also heterogeneity in the way perfectionists experience their perfectionism and their experiences with mental health, as exemplified in the accounts in the current study as well as in previous work with young perfectionists (see Molnar et al., 2023a). As such, individual counseling for perfectionistic youth will require a degree of personalization and flexibility. As demonstrated in the current work, this heterogeneity extended to young perfectionists' experiences of and reactions to the COVID-19 pandemic. Consequently, clinicians should take additional care in unpacking the idiographic ways in which individual clients experienced the COVID-19 pandemic in order to tailor interventions in ways that can appropriately and adequately address potential residual psychosocial impacts of the pandemic on young perfectionists.

As with any study, there are limitations of the current work worth noting. First, the present sample lacked diversity given that participants predominantly identified as white and female which limits the generalizability to more diverse populations. In addition, we do not have a direct comparison within our study to the experiences of non-perfectionists. Future research with more diverse samples focusing on how the experiences of youth who self-identify as perfectionists align with and diverge from those who do not identify as perfectionistic is needed to further understand how the mental health experiences of perfectionistic youth may be unique, particularly in the context of a global pandemic. Furthermore, the current work was not able to take an in-depth look at the protective factors that may bolster young perfectionists' ability to engage in the self-reflection exhibited by some of our participants who used the pandemic experience to work on themselves and see themselves as persons of worth outside their accomplishments. Additional research is needed to explore such factors as well as the ways that parents, teachers, coaches, and other practitioners working with perfectionistic youth can help to scaffold a more adaptive mindset in response to setbacks and times of uncertainty as well as a more positive and holistic view of the self. Further research will help to further inform the best approaches to intervention, support, and the amelioration of negative outcomes associated with perfectionism, including during times of public health crisis.

In conclusion, previous theory and empirical findings have provided initial evidence that perfectionistic youth were more vulnerable to the negative impacts of the pandemic than their non-perfectionistic peers (Flett, 2021; Flett & Hewitt, 2020; Hill & Madigan, 2022; Levine et al., 2022; Molnar et al., 2021, 2023c). The current work builds on these findings by providing additional insight into how and why some young perfectionists were struggling during the early stages of the pandemic. Our work also sheds light on the heterogeneity of experiences of young perfectionists during the pandemic, as some experienced some positive mental health effects during the early stages of the pandemic such as a change of pace and time to focus on the self, whereas others experienced poorer mental health and greater stress. Given that many young perfectionists experienced significant distress during the pandemic, it is increasingly important to provide support and strategies to ease their transition into a post-pandemic world and prepare them for other significant disruptions to their lives. Whereas the pandemic represented a heightened period of stress due to a lack of control along with elevated levels of uncertainty and disruption, it is only one of many intensely stressful situations faced by young perfectionists. Indeed, young perfectionists tend to be highly reactive to stress and commonly generate additional stress for themselves as a direct result of their exceptionally high standards that they impose upon themselves, which often results in more frequent failure experiences (Flett & Hewitt., 2022). Not surprisingly, perfectionistic youth were struggling and under a great deal of pressure before the pandemic and will continue to experience these challenges post-pandemic without greater awareness, intervention, and effective strategies.

We suggest general and universal strategies be employed with an understanding of the complexities associated with the presentation and experience of perfectionism. Targeted strategies run the risk of resistance and also of alienating youth who identify perfectionism as a core part of their identity. Consequently, some young perfectionists may interpret targeted approaches not as supports, but as direct attacks on their identity. Reinforcing desired behaviors such as submitting work within a given time period, engaging in self-care, and managing expectations are likely to be more effective than directly challenging cognitive distortions. When employing general and universal strategies, it is essential to take care not to feed into perfectionism (design the strategy or implementation such that it cannot be subsumed by the perfectionism and become a new outlet for expressing perfection) or further reinforce its expression and experience.

Bibliography

Appleton, P. R., & Hill, A. P. (2012). Perfectionism and athlete burnout in junior elite athletes: The mediating role of motivation regulations. *Journal of Clinical Sport Psychology*, 6(2), 129–145. <https://doi.org/10.1123/jcsp.6.2.129>

Blackburn, M., Methot-Jones, T., Molnar, D. S., Zinga, D., Spadafora, N., & Tacuri, N. (2022). Assessing changes to adolescent health-promoting behaviors following the onset of the COVID-19 pandemic: A multi-methods exploration of the role of within-person combinations of trait perfectionism. *Personality and Individual Differences, 189*, Article 111492. <https://doi.org/10.1016/j.paid.2021.111492>

Branquinho, C., Kelly, C., Arevalo, L., Santos, A., & Gaspar de Matos, M. (2020). "Hey, we also have something to say": A qualitative study of Portuguese adolescents' and young people's experiences under COVID-19. *Journal of Community Psychology, 48*(8), 2740–2752. <https://doi.org/10.1002/jcop.22453>

Braun, V., & Clarke, V. (2006). Using thematic analyses in psychology. *Qualitative Research in Psychology, 3*(2), 77–101. <https://doi.org/10.1191/1478088706qp063oa>

Braun, V., & Clarke, V. (2021). *Thematic analysis: A practical guide.* SAGE Publishing.

Burns, D. (1980). The perfectionists' script for self-defeat. *Psychology Today, 14*(6), 34–51.

Chang, E., Lee, A., Byeon, E., Seong, H., & Lee, M. (2016). The mediating effect of motivational types in the relationship between perfectionism and academic burnout. *Personality and Individual Differences, 89*, 202–210. <https://doi.org/10.1016/j.paid.2015.10.010>

Dang, S. S., Quesnel, D. A., Hewitt, P. L., Flett, G. L., & Deng, Z. (2019). Perfectionistic traits and self-presentation are associated with negative attitudes and concerns about seeking professional psychological help. *Clinical Psychology and Psychotherapy, 2020*, 1–9. <https://doi.org/10.1002/cpp.2450>

DeRosa, T. (2000). *Personality, help-seeking attitudes, and depression in adolescents.* [Doctoral dissertation, University of Toronto]. National Library of Canada. <https://bac-lac.on.worldcat.org/oclc/1335713048?lang=en>

Einstein, D. A., Lovibond, P. F., & Gaston, J. E. (2000). Relationship between perfectionism and emotional symptoms in an adolescent sample. *Australian Journal of Psychology, 52*(2), 89–93. <https://doi.org/10.1080/00049530008255373>

Ellis, W. E., Dumas, T. M., & Forbes, L. M. (2020). Physically isolated but socially connected: Psychological adjustment and stress among adolescents during the initial COVID-19 crisis. *Canadian Journal of Behavioural Science, 52*(3), 177–187. <https://doi.org/10.1037/cbs0000215>

Fervaha, G., Foussias, G., Takeuchi, H., Agid, O., & Remington, G. (2016). Motivational deficits in major depressive disorder: Cross-sectional and longitudinal relationships with functional impairment and subjective well-being. *Comprehensive Psychiatry, 66*(2016), 31–38. <https://doi.org/10.1016/j.comppsych.2015.12.004>

Flett, G. L. (2021). The anxiety epidemic among children and adolescents during the COVID-19 pandemic: Review, conceptualization, and recommendations for prevention and intervention. *Journal of Concurrent Disorders, 3*(3), 141–169. <https://doi.org/10.54127/POE3788>

Flett, G. L., & Hewitt, P. L. (2013). Disguised distress in children and adolescents "flying under the radar": Why psychological problems are underestimated and how schools must respond. *Canadian Journal of School Psychology, 28*(1), 12–27. <https://doi.org/10.1177/0829573512468845>

Flett, G. L., & Hewitt, P. L. (2014). A proposed framework for preventing perfectionism and promoting resilience and mental health among vulnerable children and adolescents. *Psychology in the Schools, 51*(9), 899–912. <https://doi.org/10.1002/pits.21792>

Flett, G. L., & Hewitt, P. L. (2020). The perfectionism pandemic meets COVID-19: Understanding the stress, distress, and problems in living for perfectionists during the global health crises. *Journal of Concurrent Disorders, 2*, 80–105. <https://doi.org/10.54127/AXGJ8297>

Flett, G. L., & Hewitt, P. L. (2022). *Perfectionism in childhood and adolescence: A developmental approach.* American Psychological Association.

Flett, G. L., Hewitt, P. L., Blankstein, K. R., & Gray, L. (1998). Psychological distress and the frequency of perfectionistic thinking. *Journal of Personality and Social Psychology, 75*(5), 1363–1381. <https://doi.org/10.1037/0022-3514.75.7.1363>

Flett, G. L., Hewitt, P. L., Blankstein, K. R., & Mosher, S. W. (1995). Perfectionism, life events, and depressive symptoms: A test of a diathesis-stress model. *Current Psychology, 14*, 112–137. <https://doi.org/10.1007/BF02686885>

Flett, G. L., Hewitt, P. L., Besser, A., Su, C., Vaillancourt, T., Boucher, D., Munro, Y., Davidson, L. A., & Gale, O. (2016). The Child-Adolescent Perfectionism Scale:

Development, psychometric properties, and associations with stress, distress, and psychiatric symptoms. *Journal of Psychoeducational Assessment, 34*, 634–652. <https://doi.org/10.1177/0734282916651381>

Goya Arce, A. B., & Polo, A. J. (2017). A test of the perfectionism social disconnection model among ethnic minority youth. *Journal of Abnormal Child Psychology, 45*, 1181–1193. <https://doi.org/10.1007/s10802-016-0240>

Hewitt, P. L., & Flett, G. L. (1991). Perfectionism in the self and social contexts: Conceptualization, assessment, and association with psychopathology. *Journal of Personality and Social Psychology, 60*(3), 456–470. <https://doi.org/10.1037/0022-3514.60.3.456>

Hewitt, P. L., Flett, G. L., & Mikail, S. F. (2017). *Perfectionism: A relational approach to conceptualization, assessment, and treatment.* The Guilford Press.

Hewitt, P. L., Flett, G. L., Sherry, S. B., & Caelian, C. (2006). Trait perfectionism dimensions and suicidal behavior. In T. E. Ellis (Ed.), *Cognition and suicide: Theory, research, and therapy* (pp. 215–235). <https://doi.org/10.1037/11377-010>

Hewitt, P. L., Flett, G. L., Sherry, S. B., Habke, M., Parkin, M., Lam, R. W., McMurtry, B., Ediger, E., Fairlie, P., & Stein, M. M. (2003). The interpersonal expression of perfection: Perfectionistic self-presentation and psychological distress. *Journal of Personality and Social Psychology, 84*(6), 1303–1325. <https://doi.org/10.1037/002-3514.84.6.1303>

Hewitt, P. L., Habke, A. M., Lee-Baggley, D. L., Sherry, S. B., & Flett, G. L. (2008). The impact of perfectionistic self-presentation on the cognitive, affective, and physiological experience of a clinical interview. *Psychiatry, 71*(2), 93–122. <https://doi.org/10.1521/psyc.2008.71.2.93>

Hewitt, P. L., Mikail, S. F., Flett, G. L., Tasca, G. A., Flynn, C. A., Deng, Z., Kaldas, J., Chen, C., & Hilsenroth, M. J. (2015). Psychodynamic/interpersonal group psychotherapy for perfectionism: Evaluating the effectiveness of a short-term treatment. *Psychotherapy, 52*(2), 205–217. <https://doi.org/10.1037/pst0000016>

Hill A. P., & Madigan, D. J. (2022). Perfectionism, mattering, stress, and self-regulation of home-learning of UK gifted and talented students during the COVID-19 pandemic. *Gifted and Talented International, 37*(1), 56–63. <https://doi-org/10.1080/15332276.2022.2033649>

Hill, A. P., Witcher, C. S. G., & Cowie, M. (2015). A qualitative study of perfectionism among self-identified perfectionists in sport and the performing arts. *Sport, Exercise, and Performance Psychology, 4*(4), 237–253. <https://doi.org/10.1037/spy0000041>

Iancheva, T., Rogaleva, A., Garcia-Mas, A., & Olmedilla, A. (2020). Perfectionism, mood states, and coping strategies of sports students from Bulgaria and Russia during the pandemic COVID-19. *Journal of Allied Sports Sciences, 1*, 22–38. <https://doi.org/10.37393/JASS.2020.01.2>

Jefsen, O. H., Rohde, C., Nørremark, B., & Østergaard, S. D. (2020). Editorial perspective: COVID-19 pandemic-related psychopathology in children and adolescents with mental illness. *Journal of Child Psychology and Psychiatry and Allied Disciplines, 62*(6), 798–800. <https://doi.org/10.1111/jcpp.13292>

Knowles, G., Gayer-Anderson, C., Turner, A., Dorn, L., Lam, J., Davis, S., Blakey, R., Lowis, K., Schools Working Group, Young Persons Advisory Group, Pinfold, V., Creary, N., Dyer, J., Hatch, S. L., Ploubidis, G., Bhui, K., Harding, S., & Morgan, C. (2022).

COVID-19, social restrictions, and mental distress among young people: A UK longitudinal, population-cased study. *The Journal of Child Psychology and Psychiatry*, *63*(11), 1382–1404. <https://doi.org/10.1111/jcpp.13586>

Larivière-Bastien, D., Aubuchon, O., Blondin, A., Dupont, D., Libenstein, J., Seguin, F., Tremblay, A., Zarglayoun, H., Herba, C. M., & Beauchamp, M. H. (2022). Children's perspectives on friendships and socialization during the COVID-19 pandemic: A qualitative approach. *Child Care Health and Development*, *48*(6), 1017–1030. <https://doi.org/10.1111/cch.12998>

Levine, S. L., Andrade, G., Koestner, R. (2022). A not so perfect plan: An examination of the differential influence of multidimensional perfectionism on missed and gained events during the COVID-19 pandemic. *Personality and Individual Differences*, *184*, Article 11214. <https://doi.org/10.1016/j.paid.2021.111214>

Limburg, K., Watson, H, J., Hagger, M. S., Egan, S. J. (2017). The relationship between perfectionism and psychopathology: A meta-analysis. *Journal of Clinical Psychology, 73*(10), 1301–1326. <https://doi.org/10.1002/jclp.22435>

Magson, N. R., Oar, E. L., Fardouly, J., Johnco, C. J., & Rapee, R. M. (2019). The preteen perfectionist: An evaluation of the perfectionism social disconnection model. *Child Psychiatry and Human Development, 50*(6), 960–974. <https://doi.org/10.1007/s10578-019-00897-2>

Molnar, D. S., Blackburn, M., Tacuri, N., Zinga, D., Flett, G. L., & Hewitt, P. L. (2023a). "I need to be perfect or else the world's gonna end": A qualitative analysis of adolescent perfectionists' expression and understanding of their perfectionism. *Canadian Psychology/Psychologie Canadienne*. <https://doi.org/10.1037/cap0000357>

Molnar, D. S., Blackburn, M., Zinga, D., Tacuri, N., Hewitt, P. L., & Flett, G. L. (2023b). Under pressure: Teacher perspectives and understandings of perfectionism among their students. Manuscript in preparation.

Molnar, D. S., Methot-Jones, T., Moore, J., Wade, T. J., & O'Leary, D. (2021). Perfectionistic cognitions pre-pandemic predict greater anxiety symptoms during the pandemic among emerging adults: A two-wave cross-lagged study. *Journal of Rational-Emotive Cognitive Behavioral Therapy, 40*, 474–492. <https://doi.org/10.1007/s10942-021-00423-1>

Molnar, D. S., Thai, S., Blackburn, M., Zinga, D., Flett, G. L., Hewitt, P. L. (2023c). Dynamic changes in perfectionism dimensions and psychological distress among adolescents assessed before and during the COVID-19 pandemic. *Child Development, 94*(1), 254–271. <https://doi.org/10.1111/cdev.13855>

Orben, A., Tomova, L., & Blakemore, S. J. (2020). The effects of social deprivation on adolescent development and mental health. *The Lancet Child & Adolescent Health, 4*(8), 634–640. <https://doi.org/10.1016/S2352-4642(20)30186-3>

QSR International Pty Ltd. (2020). NVivo (Version 12) [Computer software]. QSR. https://www.qstinternational.com/nvivo-qualitative-data-analysis-software/home

Raw, J. A., Waite, P., Pearcey, S., Shum, A., Patalay, P., & Creswell, C. (2021). Examining changes in parent-reported child and adolescent mental health throughout the UK's First COVID-19 national lockdown. *Journal of Child Psychology and Psychiatry, 62*(12), 1391–1401. <https://doi.org/10.1111/jcpp.13490>

Roxborough, H. M., Hewitt, P. L., Kaldas, J., Flett, G. L., Caelian, C. M., Sherry, S., & Sherry, D. L. (2012). Perfectionistic self-presentation, socially prescribed perfectionism, and suicide in youth: A test of the perfectionism social disconnection model. *Suicide & Life-Threatening Behavior, 42*(2), 217–233. <https://doi.org/10.1111/j.1943-278X.2012.00084.x>

Rozental, A. (2020). Beyond perfect? A case illustration of working with perfectionism using cognitive behavior therapy. *Journal of Clinical Psychology, 76*, 2041–2054. <https://doi.org/10.1002/jclp.23039>

Samji, H., Wu, J., Ladak, A., Vossen, C., Stewart, E., Dove, N., Long, D., & Snell, G. (2022). Review: Mental health impacts of the COVID-19 pandemic on children and youth—A systematic review. *Child and Adolescent Mental Health, 27*(2),173–189. <https://doi.org/10.1111/camh.12501>

Shafran, R., Coughtry, A., & Kothari, R. (2016). New frontiers in the treatment of perfectionism. *International Journal of Cognitive Therapy, 9*(2), 156–170. <https://doi.org/10.1521/ijct.2019.9.2.156>

Slaney, R. B., & Ashby J. S. (1996). Perfectionists: Study of a criterion group. *Journal of Counseling & Development, 74*, 393–398. <https://doi.org/10.1002/j.1556-6676.1996.tb01885>

Smith, M. M., Sherry, S. B., Ray, C., Hewitt, P. L., & Flett, G. L. (2021). Is perfectionism a vulnerability factor for depressive symptoms, a complication of depressive symptoms, or both? A meta-analytic test of 67 longitudinal studies. *Clinical Psychology Review, 84*, Article 101982. <https://doi.org/10.1016/j.cpr.2021.101982>

Smith, M. M., Sherry, S. B., Vidovic, V., Hewitt, P. L., & Flett, G. L. (2020). Why does perfectionism confer risk for depressive symptoms? A meta-analytic test of the mediating role of stress and social disconnection. *Journal of Research in Personality, 86*, Article 103954. <https://doi.org/10.1016/j.jrp.2020.103954>

Stoeber, J., & Rambow, A. (2007). Perfectionism in adolescent school students: Relations with motivation, achievement, and well-being. *Personality and Individual Differences, 42*(7), 1379–1389. <https://doi.org/10.1016/j.paid.2006.10.015>

Tasca, G. A., Mikail, S. F., & Hewitt, P. L. (2007). Group psychodynamic interpersonal therapy: Summary of a treatment model and outcomes for depressive symptoms. In M. J. Henri (Ed.), *Trends in depression research* (pp. 1–30). Nova Science.

Vaillancourt, T., Szatmari, P., Georgiades, K., & Krygsman, A. (2021). The impact of COVID-19 on the mental health of Canadian children and youth. *Facets, 6*, 1628–1648. <https://doi.org/10.1139/facets-2021-0078>

Villanti, A. C., LePine, S. E., Peasley-Miklus, C., West, J. C., Roemhildt, M., Williams, R., & Copeland, W. (2022). COVID-related distress, mental health, and substance use in adolescents and young adults. *Child and Adolescent Mental Health, 27*(2), 138–145. <https://doi.org/10.1111/camh.12550>

Wang, C., Pan, R., Wan, X., Tan, Y., Xu, L., Ho, C. S., & Ho, R. C. (2020). Immediate psychological responses and associated factors during the initial stage of the 2019 coronavirus disease (COVID-19) epidemic among the general population in China. *International Journal of Environmental Research and Public Health, 17*(5), Article 1729. <https://doi.org/10.3390/ijerph17051729>

Widnall, E., Winstone, L., Mars, B., Haworth, C. M. A. & Kidger, J. (2020). *Young people's mental health during the COVID-19 pandemic: Initial findings from a secondary school survey study in South West England.* <https://sphr.nihr.ac.uk/wp-content/uploads/2020/08/Young-Peoples-Mental-Health-during-the-COVID-19-Pandemic-Report.pdf>

Zinga, D., Bennett, S., Bomberry, M., & The Student Success Research Consortium. (2013). Consensus coding: Balancing perspectives in community-first research with an aboriginal community. *Paper presented at the ninth annual Congress of Qualitative Inquiry,* Urbana-Champaign.

· 4 ·

DISCLOSURES OF CHILD MALTREATMENT THROUGH COMPUTER-MEDIATED COMMUNICATION: A CALL TO ACTION

Olivia Leslie Holden, Annie Yun An Shiau, Shayla Chilliak, Victoria Talwar, and Shanna DeWit Williams

Introduction

Child maltreatment, defined as the abuse and neglect of children under the age of 18, is a prevalent issue worldwide and in Canada (Fallon et al., 2022; World Health Organization [WHO], 2022). Child maltreatment includes diverse behaviors such as physical, emotional, and sexual abuse; neglect; and exploitation, which may cause serious harm to children's mental and physical health and development (WHO, 2022). Specifically, child maltreatment increases the risk of negative outcomes including psychiatric disorders, poor physical health, high-risk behaviors, and suicide (Maniglio, 2009; Perez-Fuentes et al., 2013). Most survivors of child maltreatment do not disclose their experiences until adulthood (Ullman, 2003), which can increase the risk of negative outcomes later in life, including repeated victimization and chronic mental health problems (Lee et al., 2012). As such, child maltreatment has been highlighted as a public health crisis (e.g., Hailes et al., 2019).

Recently, Canadian children have experienced increased maltreatment during the COVID-19 pandemic, including heightened exposure to neglect and violence (Barboza et al., 2021; Kovler et al., 2020; Lawson et al., 2020). In Canada, the COVID-19 pandemic resulted in the closure of schools, non-essential services, and the enactment of physical distancing measures (Government of Canada, 2020), affecting over 5.7 million children (Statistics Canada, 2021).

While primary impacts of the pandemic on children and caregivers included direct health effects such as illness and morbidity (United Nations International Children's Emergency Fund [UNICEF], 2021b), children and their families also experienced secondary impacts such as economic struggles (Larmar et al., 2021; Lawson et al., 2020), stress (Lawson et al., 2020), social isolation during lockdowns (Lee et al., 2022), and disruptions to essential services (UNICEF, 2021b). These secondary impacts increased children's exposure to maltreatment, neglect, mental health difficulties, and domestic violence (Ridings et al., 2017; Russell et al., 2020). In addition, spaces that provided support and safety for maltreated children were unavailable; school, for example, often acts as a safe haven for children suffering from maltreatment at home (Bartholet, 2020), providing support, social connection, and physical nourishment (Cardoso et al., 2019).

Concurrent to the increased risk of maltreatment during the COVID-19 pandemic, children also faced unprecedented levels of isolation, an important barrier to maltreatment disclosure (Allnock & Miller, 2013; Best et al., 2021; Hawke et al., 2020, 2021). When experiencing maltreatment, many children seek help by disclosing their experiences to trusted individuals such as teachers, parents, doctors, nurses, and friends. Teachers, for example, are primary recipients of disclosures of child maltreatment and most frequently report suspected child maltreatment to authorities (e.g., Malloy et al., 2013). Due to pandemic lockdowns, restricted social connections, and school closures, children's access to disclosure recipients was severely restricted during the COVID-19 pandemic. As a result, child welfare agencies across Canada reported a dramatic decrease of 30–40% in reports of suspected child maltreatment during the first year of the pandemic (Haines & Jones, 2020; Katz et al., 2021; Powell, 2020). However, this decrease in reports was likely due to children's limited access to disclosure recipients, rather than reflecting decreased incidence of maltreatment (Powell, 2020).

Social isolation has led children to increasingly disclose maltreatment experiences online through computer-mediated communication (CMC; Haines & Jones, 2020;). CMC includes a vast array of technologies including text messaging, social media, websites, video calling (e.g., Zoom, FaceTime, etc.), and children's helpline services (i.e., Kids Help Phone). Pre-pandemic, many children were already turning toward CMC-facilitated services (e.g., phone, text, and online chat lines) both for general social communication (CommonSenseMedia, 2018; Steeves, 2014) and to disclose maltreatment (Vincent & David, 2004). During the COVID-19 pandemic, many children's support phone lines have transitioned to providing online and text-based services to improve children's access to services. For example, Kids Help Phone in Canada offers support in both English and French through phone, text, and chat-based services. Such services provide support to children on a variety of topics including bullying, abuse, emotional well-being, as well as receiving disclosures of child maltreat-ment. It is imperative that children who choose to disclose maltreatment experi-ences receive appropriate support and resources (Goodman-Brown et al., 2003).

Many factors may prevent children from disclosing maltreatment, such as perpetrator manipulation (e.g., threats, making the child believe the abuse is normal) and fear of what others will think (Allnock & Miller, 2013). Growing literature demonstrates that negative reactions to children's disclosures (e.g., not believing the victim, blaming the victim, minimizing the victim's experience, etc.) adversely affect the mental health of survivors; these negative reactions also deter future help-seeking and reinforce feelings of self-blame and isolation (Ahrens, 2006; Dworkin et al., 2019). In addition, after receiving an unsupportive or neg-ative reaction, a child is more likely to recant or not disclose the maltreatment again when questioned by social services (Malloy et al., 2007: Malloy & Lyon, 2006). Further, children who continue to experience maltreatment after disclos-ing their experiences to an adult experience significantly more psychiatric diffi-culties as adults compared to those who did not disclose, as children who disclose abuse may be blamed, disbelieved, or feel betrayed and unsupported by adults when disclosure is not followed by action to end the maltreatment (Swingle et al., 2016). On the other hand, children who receive appropriate support are better able to reframe their experience, avoid self-blame, and avoid short- and long-term mental health consequences (Briere & Jordan, 2004). It is thus crucial that children have ample opportunities to disclose maltreatment and that recipients respond supportively to ensure appropriate intervention and support for the child.

In sum, the COVID-19 pandemic saw an increased incidence of child mal-treatment, prevalent mental health struggles, social isolation, and expanded use of CMC for social connection. These combined factors led maltreated children to increasingly disclose their experiences through CMC. This chapter provides a review of the existing research on maltreatment disclosures through CMC by children (defined in this chapter as individuals under the age of 18). We first describe research conducted prior to the onset of the COVID-19 pandemic, then consider research conducted after the pandemic's onset. We conclude with a call for increased research and policies targeting CMC-facilitated disclosures, pro-viding specific recommendations for future research and policy development in this area.

Disclosures of Maltreatment via CMC: Evidence from Pre-Pandemic Literature

Child helplines and internet support communities are often an entry point for children to speak out and receive assistance, counseling, and referrals (Petrowski et al., 2021).

A review of English-language research conducted prior to the COVID-19 pandemic examining children's disclosures of maltreatment identified a total of six articles. These included two articles on disclosures via crisis phone lines (Elliot et al., 2022; Vincent & David, 2004), three articles on disclosures via text lines (Cash et al., 2020; Schwab-Reese et al., 2019; Schwab-Reese et al., 2022), and one article on disclosures via social media (Allagia & Wang, 2020). Specific study findings and their significance to children's disclosure are described below.

Phone Line Disclosures Pre-Pandemic

In Scotland, Vincent and David (2004) qualitatively analyzed all contacts received by ChildLine Scotland concerning child abuse and neglect over a 2-week period in 2001. ChildLine is a confidential phone line aimed at children and adolescents. Within the 2-week period, ChildLine received 217 calls for child abuse and neglect (Vincent & David, 2004). Callers ranged from children as young as 5 to those over 16, with 12–14 being the most common caller age (Vincent & David, 2004). Among the callers, 56% identified as female (n = 122) and 41% identified as male (n = 90) (Vincent & David, 2004). The most common concern reported was physical abuse (n = 106), followed by sexual abuse (n = 77). Neglect (n = 11) was the least common type of abuse disclosed (Vincent & David, 2004). The abuse described to counselors was often very serious, including being hit with a baseball bat (physical abuse), rape (sexual abuse), and being left alone or not fed (neglect) (Vincent & David, 2004). Often, more than one type of abuse (e.g., both physical abuse and neglect) was reported. Biological parents were the most commonly reported perpetrators; 29% were fathers, 24% were mothers, and 5% involved both parents (Vincent & David, 2004).

Of those children who discussed disclosure, the majority (79%) had previously told someone about the abuse (Vincent & David, 2004). The most common recipient of disclosure was a friend (n = 34), who children described as supportive and who offered advice (e.g., encouraging them to contact ChildLine), followed by a parent (n = 17) (Vincent & David, 2004). Some children described that they were not believed when disclosing to a parent (n = 12), especially when the alleged abuser was someone within the immediate family (Vincent & David, 2004). Twenty-six children had contact with official agencies such as police, school, or social work departments prior to calling, and experiences were also mixed (Vincent & David, 2004). While some children described the police as helpful and supportive, others felt that the police did not believe them and did not take any action (Vincent & David, 2004).

More recently, researchers in the United States examined de-identified messages that resulted in mandatory reporting to Child Protective Services (CPS) from a text-based crisis service between 2015 and 2017 (Cash et al., 2020; Schwab-Reese et al., 2019; Schwab-Reese et al., 2022). A dataset of 244 conversations was analyzed qualitatively and quantitatively, resulting in three separate studies with similar findings to Vincent and David (2004) (Cash et al., 2019; Schwab-Reese et al., 2019; Schwab-Reese et al., 2022). The age of children who contacted the text line ranged from 7 to 17 years (M = 14). Most children reported abuse from their mother (50%, n = 121) and/or father (46.7%, n = 113) (Cash et al., 2020; Schwab-Reese et al., 2019; Schwab-Reese et al., 2022). Again, the most common type of abuse disclosed was physical abuse (70.9%, n = 173), followed by psychological abuse (56.6%, n = 138), sexual abuse (20.9%, n = 51), and least commonly, neglect (10.7%, n = 26) (Cash et al., 2020; Schwab-Reese et al., 2019; Schwab-Reese et al., 2022). Children often reported more than one type of abuse (average types of abuse reported = 1.59), with 92.8% of children indicating that abuse was recurrent (Cash et al., 2020; Schwab-Reese et al., 2019; Schwab-Reese et al., 2022). Concurrent with the discussion of experienced abuse, many children reported mental health difficulties, including suicidal ideation (22.5%, n = 55), depression (11.9%, n = 29), self-harm (11.9%, n = 29), anxiety (9%, n = 22), and stress (8.6%, n = 21) (Schwab-Reese et al., 2019).

In a content analysis of children's text conversation with the service, the authors found that more than half of the children explicitly identified their experience as abuse and 44% disclosed the experienced maltreatment in their initial text message to the text service (Schwab-Reese et al., 2019). The authors concluded that young victims are actively seeking venues to talk about their experiences of maltreatment. As such, it is imperative that staff working in CMC-based crisis services (e.g., online chat forums) be well-trained in supportive practices to ensure a safe and positive experience (Schwab-Reese et al., 2019).

Schwab-Reese and colleagues also examined children's disclosures prior to reaching out to the text line (e.g., disclosures to peers, parents, and formal services such as police or child protection; 2022). Among the 168 conversations where children were asked if they had previously reached out for help, 20% (n = 28) had not, whereas 80% (n = 140) had (Schwab-Reese et al., 2022). Those who had sought help previously identified friends or intimate partners (n = 53), parents (n = 33), and other family members (n = 28) as primary recipients of disclosure (Schwab-Reese et al., 2022). Formal services, including mental health providers (n = 22), police (n = 16), school personnel (n = 19), and CPS (n = 10), were also reported as recipients of disclosure (Schwab-Reese et al., 2022). The authors further examined children's perception of formal systems of support. Overall, children were more comfortable disclosing to school personnel (e.g., teacher or school counselor) than with CPS or the police (Schwab-Reese et al., 2022). Many children indicated that they were afraid of the services or reported previous unpleasant experiences (e.g., services were ineffective, or children were not believed) (Schwab-Reese et al., 2022). For example, many children told the counselor that CPS had been contacted, but limited action was taken, and some believed the police would not care about their situation (Schwab-Reese et al., 2022). The authors concluded that most children are actively seeking help by disclosing maltreatment, and despite negative experiences with formal services, they are willing to make another attempt through CMC-based resources (Schwab-Reese et al., 2022).

Lastly, anonymous data collected from the National Sexual Assault Online Hotline (NSAOH), a U.S.-based free and confidential crisis hotline, found similar results among victims of child sexual abuse (Elliot et al., 2022). Elliot et al. (2022) examined 224 transcripts of session assessments between NSAOH staff and children who disclosed child sexual abuse from 2015 to 2017. Among the callers, 64% identified as female, the majority reported experiencing sexual assault (50%) or rape (44%), and 66% reported the event was ongoing (i.e., had occurred more than one time) (Elliot et al., 2022). In addition, 44% of contacts were about an event that happened within the last week (Elliot et al., 2022). Similar to the findings from the studies detailed above (Cash et al., 2020; Schwab-Reese et al., 2019; Schwab-Reese et al., 2022; Vincent & David, 2004), a parent was the most frequent perpetrator (60%), followed by a sibling (10%), an uncle (9%), and a cousin (8%) (Elliot et al., 2022).

Like the other crisis services, staff asked the child if they had previously disclosed their sexual abuse to anyone (Elliot et al., 2022). Many children disclosed the abuse to a family member (66%), including non-offending parents, and less frequently to friends (17%) or teachers (6%) (Elliot et al., 2022). Overall, most reactions to children's disclosures were negative (73%), mostly in the context of family members' reactions to disclosure (Elliot et al., 2022). Notably, 49% of non-family reactions and 50% of formal support (e.g., police, medical providers) were negative as well (Elliot et al., 2022). Negative reactions included dismissal, not believing the child, reacting with violence, and blaming the victim (Elliot et al., 2022). Only 14% of reactions were positive, with the majority of positive reactions coming from non-family members (e.g., friends, intimate partners) (Elliot et al., 2022). Positive reactions included emotional support, belief, and providing/encouraging children to seek counseling or formal support services (Elliot et al., 2022). The authors concluded that protocols for anonymous hotlines must continue to be improved to provide children with a safe space for disclosing sexual abuse (Elliot et al., 2022).

Overall, research from text and phone lines prior to the pandemic demonstrates that many children are seeking help through these services. For most children (66–80%), CMC-facilitated services are usually not their first attempt at disclosure; rather, they often turn to these services following negative experiences with formal services (Elliot et al., 2022; Schwab-Reese et al., 2022; Vincent & David, 2004). Less children (20–34%) turned to these services as their first time talking about experiences of maltreatment (Elliot et al., 2022; Schwab-Reese et al., 2022; Vincent & David, 2004). Regardless, young callers and texters disclose serious, repeated, and ongoing forms of maltreatment through CMC-facilitated services (Elliot et al., 2022; Schwab-Reese et al., 2022; Vincent & David, 2004), highlighting the significance of such services for child maltreatment researchers and policy makers alike. Alarmingly, no research prior to the COVID-19 pandemic examined the disclosure of child maltreatment through the Kids Help Phone or other CMC-facilitated crisis services in Canada.

Social Media Disclosure Pre-pandemic

In addition to phone and chat helplines, social media has also acted as a platform for children to disclose maltreatment and for adults to speak about maltreatment they experienced as a child. For example, the #MeToo movement began on social media in late 2017 (Rhode, 2019) to raise awareness about and combat sexual harassment and assault, encouraging survivors to share their experiences in order to expose the prevalence of such experiences (Alaggia & Wang, 2020). Alaggia and Wang (2020) analyzed 93 tweets and 78 Reddit posts from September and October 2018 during the #MeToo movement. The authors identified several themes regarding retrospective disclosures of childhood sexual abuse through social media. For instance, they found that social media acted as a prompt to encourage disclosure and that many adults were not aware that their prior childhood experiences constituted assault/abuse until hearing the experiences of others (Alaggia & Wang, 2020). Importantly, this highlights the increasing awareness of what constitutes maltreatment for children to accurately name their experiences and seek help. Alaggia and Wang (2020) further concluded that social media is becoming an option for disclosing and potentially healing from past sexual abuse and assault. While many posts included in this study were retrospective disclosures by adults, some posts were notably made by individuals under the age of 18; the results therefore shed light on the impact of #MeToo on social media disclosure across age groups. While the researchers conducting this study were located in the United States, the social media posts analyzed could have originated from any English-speaking user; while no data exists pertaining specifically to Canadians' social media disclosures during #MeToo, the similarity of the social media landscape in Canada and the United States suggests the results could apply to Canadian as well as American populations.

Disclosures of Maltreatment via CMC During and Following the COVID-19 Pandemic

A literature search was conducted by the authors in July 2022. Two empirical research studies were identified which examined children's CMC disclosures following the pandemic.

Phone Line Disclosures After March 2020

Petrowski et al. (2021) collected data from Child Helpline International and examined media reports to understand changes in reports of violence against children in the early months of the pandemic. Data submitted by 48 helplines across 45 countries, excluding Canada, saw an overall increase in number of contacts for any reason in the first six months of 2020 compared to 2019 (Petrowski et al., 2021). However, when specifically examining calls to report violence, a 17% decrease in contact during the second quarter of 2020 (i.e., peak of the pandemic) compared to the second quarter of 2019 was reported (Petrowski et al., 2021). Similar findings were identified by the authors' media search.

Although media articles documented an increase in total number of calls to helplines across the world, including Canada, the findings specifically examining calls about child abuse were less consistent (Petrowski et al., 2021). Evidence for increased calls to helplines regarding child abuse were identified in countries including France (34% increase of calls from minors in a dangerous situation during the first three weeks of confinement), India (over 92,000 calls received requesting protection from violence in the first 11 days of lockdown), and the United Kingdom (over 5,000 calls from adults concerned about safety of a child in March 2020) (Petrowski et al., 2021). On the other hand, reporting of violence against children to hotlines has decreased in 19 states in the U.S., where California saw a 60% decline in child abuse hotline calls during the first week of school closure (Petrowski et al., 2021). The authors concluded that spikes in calls likely reflected children seeking general COVID-19-related information, but the decline in calls regarding abuse is alarming. This may indicate that some children are not able to safely reach out for help during the lockdown (e.g., confined at home with their abusers) (Petrowski et al., 2021). However, Petrowski et al. (2021) only compared the quantity of calls immediately before and after March 2020, and did not qualitatively examine the content of the calls (e.g., what type of abuse, have you told someone) and the callers (e.g., age, gender).

We also identified evidence from gray literature indicating increased use of CMC during the COVID-19 pandemic to disclose child maltreatment. Gray literature is defined as research produced and published outside of traditional academic venues, for instance organizational reports, working papers, and government documents.

Statistics from Kids Help Phone, for instance, show a 400% increase in calls during the early months of the pandemic (Haines & Jones, 2020). Similarly, Tel-Jeunes, an online chat and phone service for children in Quebec, saw a 30% increase in demand for help during March 2020 (Lecomte, 2020).

Social Media Disclosure After March 2020

Babvey and colleagues (2021) analyzed Twitter and Reddit posts from users from the U.S. between January 2019 and July 2020. The analysis of Twitter data indicated a significant increase in abusive content generated during the time of stay-at-home restrictions (Babvey et al., 2021). However, only individual's exposure to hateful content on the internet (e.g., cyberbullying), not disclosure of such experiences, were analyzed (Babvey et al., 2021). Analysis of Reddit data provided more insight into disclosures of individual experiences. The authors found that violence-related subreddits were among the topics with the highest growth after the COVID-19 outbreak and abuse-related subreddits were among those with the highest activity growth after stay-at-home orders were enacted in March 2020 (Babvey et al., 2021). Overall, the growth in testimonials of abuse was higher than the growth in posts about other sensitive topics, including mental health (Babvey et al., 2021). It is important to note, however, that the age of these Reddit users and subreddits related specifically to child maltreatment were not examined. Therefore, the study's findings, although insightful, are not conclusive of increases in child maltreatment during the pandemic.

Call to Action: A Way Forward

The research community has a critical role to play in helping reduce child maltreatment by increasing understanding of when, how, and why children disclose maltreatment experiences, as well as what happens after their disclosure. The present chapter aimed to review existing literature on children's disclosure of maltreatment via CMC, both prior to and following the onset of the COVID-19 pandemic. We identified a few pre-pandemic studies, including research conducted on Scottish and American children's experiences with help phone and text line services (Cash et al., 2020; Schwab-Reese et al., 2019; Schwab-Reese et al., 2022; Vincent & David, 2004). One study, which examined data collected in the early months of the pandemic, was found (Petrowski et al., 2021). Petrowski et al. (2021) believed a decline in calls specifically to report violence against children is an alarming indication that some children may have more difficulties safely accessing CMC services during the lockdown. We did not find any empirical research on Canadian children's experiences disclosing maltreatment via Kids

Help Phone or any other phone or chat line. Given the increase in demand for and use of children's helpline services in Canada reported by gray literature (Haines & Jones, 2020; Ireland, 2023; Powell, 2020), it is crucial that disclosures through the Kids Help Phone in Canada be examined in more detail.

Further, we identified one empirical research study which examined subreddit disclosures prior to the COVID-19 pandemic (Allagia & Wang, 2020) and another following COVID-19 stay-at-home orders (Babvey et al., 2021). Although the articles may have included some content posted by children, the age of these Reddit posters were not able to be examined, and COVID-19 data collected by Babvey and colleagues (2021) did not examine subreddits specific to child maltreatment. Thus, there has been no research study conducted to date specifically examining children's disclosures of maltreatment through social media prior to or after the beginning of the COVID-19 pandemic. This is especially alarming given that the pandemic has led to increased rates of child maltreatment and the use of CMC for disclosure of maltreatment (Barboza et al., 2021; Haines & Jones, 2020; Katz et al., 2021; Kovler et al., 2020; Lawson et al., 2020).

Research Recommendations

Importantly, research should examine the demographics and experiences of children who reach out to crisis phone and text lines throughout the world, and specifically within Canada, in the present-day context that has shifted considerably since the onset of the COVID-19 pandemic. Research is needed to clarify the specific maltreatment experiences leading children to contact helplines and other CMC services, as well as basic demographics of children accessing such services (e.g., age, gender, race), similar to pre-pandemic research in Scotland and the United States (Cash et al., 2020; Schwab-Reese et al., 2019; Schwab-Reese et al., 2022; Vincent & David, 2004). Like these prior studies, research in Canada should also examine whether children attempted to disclose their maltreatment experiences to another individual prior to contacting the helpline or chat and whether they were met with a supportive response by the prior disclosure recipient. Given the rise in demand for helpline and chat services, it may be the case that helplines and chats are increasingly becoming children's first option for disclosure of maltreatment; further research is needed to answer this question.

Research should also focus on the specific experiences of children reaching out to help lines and chat services. This may include children's experiences with wait times for chat responses, hold times on phone lines, and whether they felt the response was supportive. Given some findings supporting that CMC disclosures rose during the pandemic while reports to CPS decreased (e.g., Haines & Jones, 2020), it is also likely that children are contacting such services anonymously. Research is needed to examine whether such services encourage children to share identifying information and to consider how CMC services can better facilitate the triage and referral of children's disclosures for investigation by formal services. It is also important to better understand where children learn about CMC services to disclose maltreatment and barriers and facilitators to children accessing such services.

Future research should incorporate data collection from more diverse CMC platforms, including social media. Although most social media platforms require users to be at least 13 years old, many popular sites do not verify users' age upon registration (e.g., Discord) or could be easily bypassed by entering a fake birthday (e.g., YouTube, TikTok, etc.). Currently, articles examining social media disclosures mostly place a focus on retrospective or current adult disclosures (e.g., Alaggia & Wang, 2020). No study to date has examined children's disclosures of maltreatment on social media. Now more than ever, children use social media to discuss difficult topics. TikTok is one of the fastest rising and most popular online platforms among Canadian children (Deschamps, 2023); 54% of Canadian children between the ages of 9–17 years old have a TikTok account (MediaSmarts, 2022). This platform contains extensive discussion of difficult topics including mental health and abuse; for example, at the time this chapter was written, the hashtag #CSASurvivor (Child Sexual Abuse Survivor) has over 568.4 million views, #ChildhoodTraumaSurvivor has over 72.4 million views and #CASurvivor (Child Abuse Survivor) has over 9.8 million views.

The lack of research on this topic may be due to the anonymity of the internet and the inability to confirm the ages of those posting on social media. However, research conducted with data from social media is not without its controversies. Many researchers call into question the ethics of utilizing public social media posts in research projects, as these individuals have not consented to their information being used for research (e.g., Hunter et al., 2018). The ethical boundaries of such research may be even more contested when social media posters are children. Regardless, given the popularity of such platforms to discuss abuse and maltreatment, it is important for researchers to find a way to examine data from social media to understand ongoing shifts in how children are disclosing.

It is also important to better understand the factors that influence children's decisions to disclose through CMC, including mental health factors. For example, do children turn to CMC-facilitated services in times of heightened loneliness, isolation or other mental health difficulties? Why do they prefer to disclose via CMC rather than another outlet, if available? Given previous findings that most children reporting through CMC had already disclosed to another person (e.g., Elliot et al., 2022), it is also important to examine whether children who turn to CMC exhibit traits of resilience that allow them to persevere in their search for help. Developmental factors such as age should also be explored. As younger children may have limited access to and knowledge of how to use CMC devices, it is possible that CMC is not a primary choice for disclosure at a younger age. Research designs that incorporate children's voices and perspectives will also be necessary to improve our understanding of their experiences disclosing maltreatment via CMC.

Lastly, research should examine the impact of recent implementation of Artificial Intelligence (AI) in CMC chat and text services. Given the recent increase in demand for CMC phone, text, and chat lines in Canada, the Kids Help Phone has recently partnered with the Vector Institute, an organization for responsible AI implementation, to begin incorporating AI into their services (Ireland, 2023). This change would allow AI to detect keywords and speech patterns from children reaching out to the Kids Help Phone to help counselors better prioritize and triage chats (Ireland, 2023). Kids Help Phone states that this change will not remove the person to person contact between the child and counselor, but instead will be used to help counselors monitor key points in their discussions (Ireland, 2023). It is important to consider ethical concerns including use of AI and responsibility of individuals conducting harm and risk assessments, data ethics issues, and level of guidance in the development and implementation of this technology (Fiske et al., 2019). Research should also monitor the impact of AI on the user experience for children contacting CMC services to disclose maltreatment, as well as the experiences of counselors implementing AI to effectively support children.

Policy Recommendations

The existing CMC-facilitated crisis services, including phone and text lines, are used by many children throughout the world, specifically within Canada. Importantly, many children report negative experiences when disclosing maltreatment to informal (e.g., parents, friends) and/or formal recipients (e.g., police, CPS; Elliot et al., 2022; Schwab-Reese et al., 2022; Vincent & David, 2004). As a result, it is possible that many children are turning toward CMC-facilitated services when other methods of disclosure have failed them (Schwab-Reese et al., 2019; Schwab-Reese et al., 2022). In order for children using CMC-facilitated services to receive proper support, services should ensure that staff and volunteers are adequately trained in how to respond supportively to children's disclosures and should provide oversight to ensure that training is put into practice consistently. Given that children contacting CMC services are often also experiencing mental health difficulties (Elliot et al., 2022), an emphasis on mental health factors associated with child maltreatment should be included in training programs.

Additionally, CMC-facilitated services must also be sufficiently staffed and funded. In Vincent and David's (2004) analysis of a Scottish hotline, for example, the phone line relied on volunteers and was only able to respond to about half of incoming calls. Given that many children are reaching out to CMC-facilitated services regarding active and serious abuse (Schwab-Reese et al., 2022; Vincent & David, 2004), it is important that adequate government funding be allocated to these crisis services to support staffing and training. The use of AI in CMC support services should also continue to be monitored and considered by policymakers, specifically in terms of data security and user experience.

It is also important that CMC-facilitated services work closely with child protection organizations to deliver appropriate interventions for child maltreatment. Given that CMC-mediated disclosures may happen anonymously, it is important for such services to consult with child protection to determine appropriate ways to support children in disclosing information required to verify their identity and intervene appropriately. Developing strategies to better identify victims of maltreatment reaching out through CMC-facilitated services or platforms could result in more active intervention and prevention of child maltreatment.

Conclusion

Child maltreatment is a serious issue resulting in significant negative mental health outcomes during childhood and into adulthood. During the COVID-19 pandemic, children experienced increased risk of maltreatment, increased mental health struggles, and reduced avenues to speak about maltreatment. As such, children have turned increasingly to CMC-mediated services, such as phone lines, chat and text services, and social media, to disclose maltreatment. Concerningly, very few empirical research studies to date have examined children's maltreatment disclosures via CMC during or after the height of the COVID-19 pandemic. There is a dire need for research to better understand how and why children are increasingly disclosing maltreatment via CMC since the onset of the COVID-19 pandemic, as well as to elucidate their specific experiences with such services. This chapter puts forth a call to action for researchers and policymakers alike to increase focus on the role of CMC in children's disclosure of maltreatment. Further, we specifically recommend centering children's own perspectives in said research. In terms of policy, it is crucial that adequate funding be provided to CMC-facilitated crisis services in order to maintain a safe and positive space for children to talk about experienced maltreatment, especially when other disclosure recipients have failed them. These steps will be crucial to facilitate trauma-informed and child-centered CMC services as technologies become a growing part of everyday human lives.

Bibliography

Ahrens, C. E. (2006). Being silenced: The impact of negative social reactions on the disclosure of rape. *American Journal of Community Psychology, 38*(3–4), 263–274. <https://doi.org/10.1007/s10464-006-9069-9>

Alaggia, R., & Wang, S. (2020). "I never told anyone until the #metoo movement": What can we learn from sexual abuse and sexual assault disclosures made through social media? *Child Abuse & Neglect, 103*, Article 104312. <https://doi.org/10.1016/j.chiabu.2019.104312>

Allnock, D., & Miller, P. (2013). No one noticed, no one heard: A study of disclosures of childhood abuse. NSPCC. <https://learning.nspcc.org.uk/research-resources/2013/no-one-noticed-no-one-heard>

Babvey, P., Capela, F., Cappa, C., Lipizzi, C., Petrowski, N., & Ramirez-Marquez, J. (2021). Using social media data for assessing children's exposure to violence during the COVID-19 pandemic. *Child Abuse & Neglect, 116*, 104747. <https://doi.org/10.1016/j.chiabu.2020.104747>

Barboza, G. E., Schiamberg, L. B., & Pachl, L. (2021). A spatiotemporal analysis of the impact of COVID-19 on child abuse and neglect in the city of Los Angeles, California. *Child Abuse & Neglect, 116*, Article 04740. <https://doi.org/10.1016/j.chiabu.2020.104740>

Baron, E. J., Goldstein, E. G., & Wallace, C. T. (2020). Suffering in silence: How COVID-19 school closures inhibit the reporting of child maltreatment. *Journal of Public Economics, 190*, Article 104258. <https://doi.org/https://doi.org/10.1016/j.jpubeco.2020.104258>

Barreto, M., Victor, C., Hammond, C., Eccles, A., Richins, M. T., & Qualter, P. (2021). Loneliness around the world: Age, gender, and cultural differences in loneliness. *Personality and Individual Differences, 169*, Article 110066. <https://doi.org/10.1016/j.chiabu.2020.104740>

Bartholet, E. (2020). Homeschooling: Parent rights absolutism vs. child rights to education & protection. *Arizona Law Review, 62*(1), 1–80. <http://dx.doi.org/10.2139/ssrn.3391331>

Belsky, J. (1980). Child maltreatment: An ecological integration. *American Psychologist, 35*(4), 320–335. <https://doi.org/10.1037/0003-066X.35.4.320>

Belsky J. (1993). Etiology of child maltreatment: A developmental-ecological analysis. *Psychological Bulletin, 114*(3), 413–434. <https://doi.org/10.1037/0033-2909.114.3.413>

Best, L. A., Law, M. A., Roach, S., & Wilbiks, J. M. (2021). The psychological impact of COVID-19 in Canada: Effects of social isolation during the initial response. *Canadian Psychology/Psychologie Canadienne, 62*(1), 143–154. <https://doi.org/10.1037/cap0000254>

Briere, J., & Jordan, C. E. (2004). Violence against women: Outcome complexity and implications for assessment and treatment. *Journal of Interpersonal Violence, 19*(11), 1252–1276. <https://doi.org/10.1177/0886260504269682>

Brooks-Gunn, J., Schneider, W., & Waldfogel, J. (2013). The great recession and the risk for child maltreatment. *Child Abuse & Neglect, 37*(10), 721–729. <https://doi.org/10.1016/j.chiabu.2013.08.004>

Cardoso, S. G., Truninger, M., Ramos, V., & Augusto, F. R. (2019). School meals and food poverty: Children's views, parents' perspectives and the role of school. *Children & Society, 33*(6), 572–586. <https://doi.org/10.1111/chso.12336>

Cardy, R. E., Dupuis, A., Anagnostou, E., Ziolkowski, J., Biddiss, E. A., Monga, S., Brian, J., Penner, M., & Kushki, A. (2021). Characterizing changes in screen time during the COVID-19 pandemic school closures in Canada and its perceived impact on children with autism spectrum disorder. *Frontiers in Psychiatry, 12*, Article 702774. <https://doi.org/10.3389/fpsyt.2021.702774>

Cash, S. J., Murfree, L., & Schwab-Reese, L. (2020). "I'm here to listen and want you to know I am a mandated reporter": Understanding how text message-based crisis counselors facilitate child maltreatment disclosures. *Child Abuse & Neglect, 102*, 104414. <https://doi.org/10.1016/j.chiabu.2020.104414>

Conrad-Hiebner, A., & Byram, E. (2020). The temporal impact of economic insecurity on child maltreatment: A systematic review. *Trauma, Violence & Abuse, 21*(1), 157–178. <https://doi.org/10.1177/1524838018756122>

Coulton, C. J., Crampton, D. S., Irwin, M., Spilsbury, J. C., & Korbin, J. E. (2007). How neighborhoods influence child maltreatment: A review of the literature and alternative pathways. *Child Abuse & Neglect, 31*(11), 1117–1142. <https://doi.org/https://doi.org/10.1016/j.chiabu.2007.03.023>

Davidson Arad, B., McLeigh, J. D., & Katz, C. (2020). Perceived collective efficacy and parenting competence: The roles of quality of life and hope. *Family Process, 59*(1), 273–287. <https://doi.org/10.1111/famp.12405>

Deschamps, T. (2023, March 9). TikTok is the fastest growing social media app in Canada— but least trusted: Report. *Global News.* <https://globalnews.ca/news/9538635/tiktok-trust-canada-social-media-apps/>

Dworkin, E. R., Brill, C. D., & Ullman, S. E. (2019). Social reactions to disclosure of interpersonal violence and psychopathology: A systematic review and meta-analysis. *Clinical Psychology Review, 72*, Article 101750. <https://doi.org/10.1016/j.cpr.2019.101750>

Elliott, S. A., Goodman, K. L., Bardwell, E. S., & Mullin, T. M. (2022). Reactions to the disclosure of intrafamilial childhood sexual abuse: Findings from the National Sexual Assault Online Hotline. *Child Abuse & Neglect, 127*, Article 105567. <https://doi.org/10.1016/j.chiabu.2022.105567>

Ellis, W. E., Dumas, T. M., & Forbes, L. M. (2020). Physically isolated but socially connected: Psychological adjustment and stress among adolescents during the initial COVID-19 crisis. *Canadian Journal of Behavioural Science / Revue canadienne des sciences du comportement, 52*(3), 177–187. <https://doi.org/10.1037/cbs0000215>

Fallon, B., Joh-Carnella, N., Trocmé, N., Esposito, T., Hélie, S., & Levebvre, R. (2022). Major findings from the Canadian incidence study of reported child abuse and neglect. *International Journal on Child Maltreatment, 5*, 1–17. <https://doi.org/10.1007/s42448-021-00110-9>

Favotto, L., Michaelson, V., Pickett, W., & Davison, C. (2019). The role of family and computer-mediated communication in adolescent loneliness. *PLoS ONE, 14*(6), Article e0214617. <https://doi.org/10.1371/journal.pone.0214617>

Finkel, M. A., & DeJong, A. R. (1994). Medical findings in child sexual abuse. In R. M. Reece (Ed.), *Child abuse: Medical diagnosis and management* (pp. 185–247). Lea & Febiger.

Fiske, A., Henningsen, P., & Buyx, A. (2019). Your robot therapist will see you now: Ethical implications of embodied artificial intelligence in psychiatry, psychology, and psychotherapy. *Journal of Medical Internet Research, 21*(5), Article e13216. <https://doi:10.2196/13216>

Goodman-Brown, T. B., Edelstein, R. S., Goodman, G. S., Jones, D. P. H., & Gordon, D. S. (2003). Why children tell: A model of children's disclosure of sexual abuse. *Child Abuse & Neglect, 27*(5), 525–540. <https://doi.org/10.1016/s0145-2134(03)00037-1>

Government of Canada. (2020, April 3). Community-based measures to mitigate the spread of coronavirus disease (COVID-19) in Canada. <https://www.canada.ca/en/public-health/services/diseases/2019-novel-coronavirus-infection/health-professionals/public-health-measures-mitigate-covid-19.html>

Hailes, H. P., Yu, R., Danese, A., & Fazel, S. (2019). Long-term outcomes of childhood sexual abuse: An umbrella review. *The Lancet Psychiatry, 6*(10), 830–839. <https://doi.org/10.1016/s2215-0366(19)30286-x>

Haines, A., & Jones, A. M. (2020, May 5). Advocates concerned child abuse going unreported with schools closed. *CTV News.* <https://www.ctvnews.ca/canada/advocates-concerned-child-abuse-going-unreported-with-schools-closed-1.4926814>

Hawke, L. D., Barbic, S. P., Voineskos, A., Szatmari, P., Cleverley, K., Hayes, E., Relihan, J., Daley, M., Courtney, D., Cheung, A., Darnay, K., & Henderson, J. L. (2020). Impacts of COVID-19 on youth mental health, substance use, and well-being: A rapid survey of clinical and community samples. *Canadian Journal of Psychiatry, 65*(10), 701–709. <https://doi.org/10.1177/0706743720940562>

Hawke, L. D., Hayes, E., Darnay, K., & Henderson, J. (2021). Mental health among transgender and gender diverse children: An exploration of effects during the COVID-19 pandemic. *Psychology of Sexual Orientation and Gender Diversity, 8*(2), 180–187. <https://doi.org/10.1037/sgd0000467>

Hawkley, L. C., & Capitanio, J. P. (2015). Perceived social isolation, evolutionary fitness and health outcomes: A lifespan approach. *Philosophical Transactions of the Royal Society of London, Series B, Biological Sciences, 370*(1669), Article 20140114. <https://doi.org/10.1098/rstb.2014.0114>

Hunter, R. F., Gough, A., O'Kane, N., McKeown, G., Fitzpatrick, A., Walker, T., McKinley, M., Lee, M., & Kee, F. (2018). Ethical issues in social media research for public health. *American Journal of Public Health, 108*(3), 343–348. <https://doi.org/10.2105/AJPH.2017.304249>

Ireland, N. (2023, July 5). Kids Help Phone seeking help from AI tech to meet demand for mental health support. *CTV News Toronto.* <https://toronto.ctvnews.ca/kids-help-phone-seeking-help-from-ai-tech-to-meet-demand-for-mental-health-support-1.6467525>

Katz, I., Katz, C., Andresen, S., Bérubé, A., Collin-Vezina, D., Fallon, B., Fouché, A., Haffejee, N. M., Muñoz, P. Filho, S. R. P., Tarabulsy, G., Truter, E., Varela, N., & Wekerle, C. (2021). Child maltreatment reports and child protection service responses during covid-19: Knowledge exchange among Australia, Brazil, Canada, Colombia, Germany, Israel, and South Africa. *Child Abuse & Neglect, 116*, Article 105078. <https://doi.org/10.1016/j.chiabu.2021.105078>

Kovler, M. L., Ziegfeld, S., Ryan, L. M., Goldstein, M. A., Gardner, R., Garcia, A. V., & Nasr, I. W. (2021). Increased proportion of physical child abuse injuries at a level I pediatric trauma center during the Covid-19 pandemic. *Child Abuse & Neglect, 116*, Article 104756. <https://doi.org/10.1016/j.chiabu.2020.104756>

Larmar, S., Sunuwar, M., Sherpa, H., Joshi, R., & Jordan, L. P. (2021). Strengthening community engagement in Nepal during COVID-19: Community-based training and development to reduce child labour. *Asia Pacific Journal of Social Work and Development, 31*(1–2), 23–30. <https://doi.org/10.1080/02185385.2020.1833749>

Lawson, M., Piel, M. H., & Simon, M. (2020). Child maltreatment during the COVID-19 pandemic: Consequences of parental job loss on psychological and physical abuse towards children. *Child Abuse & Neglect, 110*, Article 104709. <https://doi.org/https://doi.org/10.1016/j.chiabu.2020.104709>

Lecomte, A. M. (2020, March 31). Tel-jeunes et LigneParents sont débordés en raison de la COVID-19. *Radio-Canada.* <https://ici.radio-canada.ca/nouvelle/1689947/tel-jeunes-ligneparents-covid19-quebec-aide-detresse-famille-suicide>

Lee, A., Coles, J., Lee, S. J., & Kulkarni, J. (2012). Women survivors of child abuse—Don't ask, don't tell. *Australian Family Physician, 41(11)*, 903–906.

Lee, S. J., Ward, K. P., Lee, J. Y., Rodriguez, C. (2022). Parental social isolation and child maltreatment risk during the COVID-19 pandemic. *Journal of Family Violence, 37*, 813–824. <https://doi.org/10.1007/s10896-020-00244-3>

Maguire-Jack, K. (2014). Multilevel investigation into the community context of child maltreatment. *Journal of Aggression, Maltreatment & Trauma, 23*(3), 229–248. <https://doi.org/10.1080/10926771.2014.881950>

Malloy, L. C., Brubacher, S. P., & Lamb, M. E. (2013). "Because she's one who listens": Children discuss disclosure recipients in forensic interviews. *Child Maltreatment, 18*(4), 245–251. <https://doi.org/10.1177/1077559513497250>

Malloy, L. C., & Lyon, T. D. (2006). Caregiver support and child sexual abuse: Why does it matter? *Journal of Child Sexual Abuse, 15*(4), 97–103. <https://doi.org/10.1300/J070v15n04_06>

Malloy, L. C., Lyon, T. D., & Quas, J. A. (2007). Filial dependency and recantation of child sexual abuse allegations. *Journal of the American Academy of Child and Adolescent Psychiatry, 46*(2), 162–170. <https://doi.org/10.1097/01.chi.0000246067.77953.f7>

Maniglio, R. (2009). The impact of child sexual abuse on health: A systematic review of reviews. *Clinical Psychology Review, 29*(7), 647–657. <https://doi.org/10.1016/j.cpr.2009.08.003>

Marani, I. N., Subarkah, A., & Wijayanto, A. (2020). The use of computer-mediated communication (CMC) In distance learning during covid-19 pandemic: Pros and cons. *Proceedings of the 6th International Conference on Social and Political Sciences (ICOSAPS 2020)*, 95–102. <https://doi.org/10.2991/assehr.k.201219.015>

MediaSmarts. (2022). *Young Canadians in a Wireless World, Phase IV: Life Online.* <https://mediasmarts.ca/sites/default/files/publication-report/full/life-online-report-en-final-11-22.pdf>

Molnar, B. E., Goerge, R. M., Gilsanz, P., Hill, A., Subramanian, S. V., Holton, J. K., Duncan, D. T., Beatriz, E. D., & Beardslee, W. R. (2016). Neighborhood-level social processes and substantiated cases of child maltreatment. *Child Abuse & Neglect, 51*, 41–53. <https://doi.org/https://doi.org/10.1016/j.chiabu.2015.11.007>

People for Education (2021, October 5). *Comparing School COVID-19 Policies Across Canada.* <https://peopleforeducation.ca/our-work/comparing-school-covid-19-policies-across-canada/>

Perez-Fuentes, G., Olfson, M., Villegas, L., Morcillo, C., Wang, S., & Blanco, C. (2013). Prevalence and correlates of child sexual abuse: A national study. *Comprehensive Psychiatry, 54*(1), 16–27. <https://doi.org/10.1016/j.comppsych.2012.05.010>

Petrowski, N., Cappa, C., Pereira, A., Mason, H., & Daban, R. A. (2021). Violence against children during COVID-19: Assessing and understanding change in use of helplines. *Child Abuse & Neglect, 116*, Article 104757. <https://doi.org/https://doi.org/10.1016/j.chiabu.2020.104757>

Powell, B. (2020, April 27). *Kids help calls are soaring amid COVID-19, but not criminal reports. Are we in the dark on child abuse?.* The Star. <https://www.thestar.com/news/canada/2020/04/27/kids-help-calls-are-soaring-amid-covid-19-but-not-criminal-reports-are-we-in-the-dark-on-child-abuse.html.>

Proulx, K., Lenzi-Weisbecker, R., Rachel, R., Hackett, K., Cavallera, V., Daelmans, B., & Dua, T. (2021). Responsive caregiving, opportunities for early learning, and children's safety and security during COVID-19: A rapid review. *MedRxiv.* <https://doi.org/10.1101/2021.02.10.21251507>

Public Health Ontario. (2021). *Negative Impacts of Community-based Public Health Measures on Children, Adolescents and Families During the COVID-19 Pandemic: Update.* <https://www.publichealthontario.ca/-/media/documents/ncov/he/2021/01/rapid-review-neg-impacts-children-youth-families.pdf?la=en>

Rhode, D. L. (2019). #metoo: why now: what next. Duke Law Journal, 69(2), 377–428.

Ridings, L. E., Beasley, L. O. & Silovsky, J. F. (2017). Consideration of risk and protective factors for families at risk for child maltreatment: An intervention approach. *Journal of Family Violence, 32*, 179–188. <https://doi.org/10.1007/s10896-016-9826-y>

Rodriguez, C. M., Lee, S. J., Ward, K. P., & Pu, D. F. (2021). The perfect storm: Hidden risk of child maltreatment during the Covid-19 pandemic. *Child Maltreatment, 26*(2), 139–151. <https://doi.org/10.1177/1077559520982066>

Russell, B. S., Hutchison, M., Tambling, R., Tomkunas, A. J., & Horton, A. L. (2020). Initial challenges of caregiving during COVID-19: Caregiver burden, mental health, and the parent–child relationship. *Child Psychiatry & Human Development, 51*, 671–682. <https://doi.org/10.1007/s10578-020-01037-x>

Schwab-Reese, L., Kanuri, N., & Cash, S. (2019). Child maltreatment disclosure to a text messaging-based crisis service: Content analysis. *JMIR mHealth and uHealth, 7*(3), Article e11306. <https://doi.org/10.2196/11306>

Schwab-Reese, L. M., Cash, S. J., Lambert, N. J., & Lansford, J. E. (2022). "They aren't going to Do jack shit": Text-based crisis service users' perceptions of seeking child maltreatment-related support from formal systems. *Journal of Interpersonal Violence, 37*(19–20). <https://doi.org/10.1177/08862605211043577>

Seddighi, H., Salmani, I., Javadi, M. H., & Seddighi, S. (2021). Child abuse in natural disasters and conflicts: A systematic review. *Trauma, Violence, & Abuse, 22*(1), 176–185. <https://doi.org/10.1177/1524838019835973>

Statistics Canada. (2019a). *A portrait of Canadian youth: March 2019 updates.* <https://www150.statcan.gc.ca/n1/en/catalogue/11-631-X2019003>

Statistics Canada. (2019b). *Census profile, 2016 census.* <https://www12.statcan.gc.ca/census-recensement/2016/dp-pd/prof/index.cfm?Lang=E>

Statistics Canada. (2020, July). *Impacts of COVID-19 on Canadian families and children.* <https://www150.statcan.gc.ca/n1/daily-quotidien/200709/dq200709a-eng.htm>

Statistics Canada (2021). *School closures and COVID-19: Interactive tool.* <https://www150.statcan.gc.ca/n1/pub/71-607-x/71-607-x2021009-eng.htm>

Steeves, V. (2014). *Young Canadians in a wired world, phase III: Trends and recommendations.* MediaSmarts. <https://mediasmarts.ca/sites/default/files/publication-report/full/ycwwiii_trends_recommendations_fullreport.pdf>

Swingle, J. M., Tursich, M., Cleveland, J. M., Gold, S. N., Tolliver, S. F., Michaels, L., Kupperman-Caron, L. N., Garcia-Larrieu, M., & Sciarrino N. A. (2016). Childhood disclosure of sexual abuse: Necessary but not necessarily sufficient. *Child Abuse & Neglect, 62*, 10–18. <https://doi.org/10.1016/j.chiabu.2016.10.009>

Ullman, S. E. (2003). Social reactions to child sexual abuse disclosures: A critical review. *Journal of Child Sexual Abuse, 12*(1), 89–121. <https://doi.org/10.1300/J070v12n01_05>

UNICEF. (2020). *COVID-19 and its implications for protecting children online.* <https://www.unicef.org/documents/covid-19-and-implications-protecting-children-online>.

UNICEF. (2021a). *Children are at increased risk of harm online during the global COVID-19 pandemic, says UNICEF.* <https://www.unicef.org/venezuela/en/press-releases/children-are-increased-risk-harm-online-during-global-covid-19-pandemic-says-unicef>

UNICEF. (2021b). *Primary and secondary impacts of the COVID-19 pandemic on children in Ghana.* <https://www.unicef.org/ghana/media/3486/file/Effects%20of%20COVID-19%20on%20Women%20and%20Children%20in%20Ghana%20(II).pdf>

Vincent, S. & Daniel, B. (2004). An analysis of children and young people's calls to ChildLine about abuse and neglect: A study for the Scottish Child Protection Review. *Child Abuse Review, 13*, 158–171. <https://doi.org/10.1002/car.840>

World Health Organization (2021). *Child maltreatment.* <https://www.who.int/news-room/fact-sheets/detail/child-maltreatment>

Wu, Q., & Xu, Y. (2020). Parenting stress and risk of child maltreatment during the COVID-19 pandemic: A family stress theory-informed perspective. *Developmental Child Welfare, 2*(3), 180–196. <https://doi.org/10.1177/2516103220967937>

· 5 ·

RECOMMENDATIONS TO MITIGATE FUTURE PANDEMIC IMPACTS ON HEALTH PROFESSIONS EDUCATION: LESSONS LEARNED DURING THE COVID-19 PANDEMIC

Kelly Lackie, Neda Alizadeh, Mark Embrett, Simon Field, Jennifer Lane, Marion Brown, Diane MacKenzie, Bright Huo, Kathleen MacMillan, and Ruth Martin-Misener

Introduction

The COVID-19 pandemic created unprecedented and ongoing health, economic, and social challenges globally, including disruption to health professions education and health systems (Alsoufi et al., 2020). On March 17, 2020, public health measures in Nova Scotia, Canada resulted in the immediate suspension of skills-based learning (SBL) for Dalhousie University Faculty of Health (FoH) and Medicine (FoM) students. The FoH comprises a number of schools—Health and Human Performance, Health Administration, Communication Sciences and Disorders, Nursing, Occupational Therapy, Physiotherapy, Social Work, the QEII/Dalhousie School of Health Sciences (sonographers, nuclear medicine technologists, radiological technologists, respiratory therapists and medical lab technologists), one college (Pharmacy), and one standalone program (the Clinical Vision Science Program located at the IWK Health Center). There are also a number of diploma and certificate programs that are part of the FoH schools/college (Dalhousie University Faculty of Health, 2023). Only those students who held a license to practice in their respective professions (e.g., medical and pharmacy residents) were able to continue clinical practice. For the remainder of students who did not hold a license to practice, the suspension of SBL meant placing the continuation of their programs on hold for the foreseeable future. Suspensions only began to ease between June and August 2020 (Merritt, 2020a; 2020b), with strict adherence to public health guidelines (Chief Medical Officer of Health, 2021).

Due to the diversity of programs in the FoH and FoM, we use the term SBL to capture practical skills acquisition, including communication, hands-on, decision-making, and problem-solving skills, that occur in various settings (clinical/fieldwork, simulation) and disciplines. This study aimed to determine the impact of FoH/FoM pandemic-related curricular changes to SBL during the first wave of the pandemic (March to August 2020) and capitalize on what we learned to inform recommendations for student learning during future pandemics or global disasters.

At the onset of the pandemic, little evidence existed to inform decisions about the curricular changes needed to adjust to public health restrictions while preserving opportunities for students to achieve program-specific learning outcomes. Across Canada, during the first wave of the pandemic, the impact of restrictions varied. For example, the Quebec government permitted professional governing bodies to allow nursing students, with no more than one semester remaining in their program, to work in long-term care (LTC) facilities (Boshra, 2020). In British Columbia, the nursing regulatory body registered entry-level nursing students for employment in certain healthcare settings (e.g., community care) (British Columbia College of Nursing Professionals, 2020), a decision that was postulated to release registered nurses to care for higher acuity patients. To alleviate strain on the Ontario healthcare system, the Ministry of Health sought health professions students to volunteer in healthcare delivery (College of Nurses of Ontario, 2020). In Nova Scotia and New Brunswick, where Dalhousie University students pursue clinical training, students in dentistry, medicine, nursing, occupational therapy, physiotherapy, and/or social work offered volunteer services, such as grocery shopping and childcare, to frontline healthcare workers (Gorman, 2020; Smith, 2020).

To help alleviate the strain on the healthcare system, Canadian academic associations and health authorities supported proposals to rapidly teach and assess entry-to-practice competencies to expedite students' entry into their fields of practice to assist in the delivery of healthcare services during the pandemic (Cooke, 2022; Foroozan, 2020; Ontario Physiotherapy Association, 2022). Concomitantly, there was recognition that to maintain public safety, novice practitioners needed to be adequately prepared (e.g., additional training, orientation to role) (Williams et al., 2020), supervised, and supported to volunteer and/or participate in extracurricular activities in healthcare settings (Canadian Association of Schools of Nursing, 2020). Health professions students require opportunities for SBL to attain their respective entry-level competencies to practice safely in their chosen profession. The ongoing disruptions to clinical learning across waves of the pandemic raised concern among students and educators regarding how to include these students safely and appropriately in SBL (McFadden et al., 2022). The closure of clinical placements would interfere with the acquisition of clinical and interprofessional skills and impede the attainment of clinical hours required in the respective programs (Stout et al., 2021); this would create backlogs in students' ability to complete their academic program in a timely manner and restrict entry of new students to these programs, further burdening the healthcare system. Related research regarding the impact of the pandemic on students' learning in clinical settings during times when access to SBL was restricted suggests that the unprecedented challenges require an aptitude for adaptability and may offer novel opportunities for participation in SBL during a pandemic (Dedeilia et al., 2020). This study presents important information about how pandemic-related curricular changes to SBL during the first wave of the pandemic impacted student capacity to learn professional skills and proposes strategies to use when rapid curricular changes threaten to impede health professional student SBL.

Methodology

Theoretical Framework

Challenges affecting the health workforce results in obstacles to the delivery of health services and, ultimately, health systems performance (Lackie & Tomblin Murphy, 2020). Health human resources planning (HHRP) calls for examination of the composition, distribution, and behavior of healthcare providers (HCPs) that are required in the system to meet population healthcare needs (Lackie & Tomblin Murphy, 2020). Service-based HHRP (SBHHRP) (Tomblin Murphy et al., 2013), considers the competencies HCPs require to provide healthcare services (Lackie & Tomblin Murphy, 2020), positioning it as an ideal framework to explore the impact of education and training disruptions (e.g., to SBL) on health professions students who will soon enter the system.

SBHHRP allows planners to identify healthcare service needs and ways to meet them, determine the number and types of HCPs needed to provide services, and decide how best to deploy HCPs based on their scopes of practice. This study specifically focused on the production (education and training) element of the SBHHRP framework. Previous works by Tomblin Murphy (2007) and Lackie and Tomblin Murphy (2020) support the significance of this framework to investigate the impact of the pandemic on health professions education and the potential long-term consequences for the HHRP field. The research team applied the

SBHHRP framework to the findings to make recommendations about how to best address the impact of the pandemic on SBL to address the health system's capacity to respond to population healthcare needs.

Methods

Using a concurrent mixed methodological approach, qualitative (interviews/focus group) and quantitative (survey) data were collected concurrently and with equal priority (both strands of equal importance) between April and November 2021. Mixing of data occurred during interpretation, where the results from both strands were compared and/or synthesized and conclusions drawn (Creswell & Plano Clark, 2018).

Setting, Sample, and Recruitment

The study was conducted virtually and approved by the Nova Scotia Health (NSH) Research Ethics Board (REB file #1027266). NSH is the largest provincial health authority in Nova Scotia providing health services throughout 45 different facilities (Nova Scotia Health Authority, 2023). Undergraduate and graduate FoH and FoM students enrolled in entry-to-practice programs with SBL components, plus 2020 graduates of these programs were invited to participate via email and social media (e.g., Twitter (X), Facebook). Over 3000 students were enrolled in the FoH, and approximately 450 students were in the Undergraduate Medical Education (UGME) program in the FoM.

All students were invited to complete an online survey and participate in interviews and/or focus groups. Faculty members from both faculties were invited to participate in interviews and focus groups through faculty listservs. NSH clinical placement managers responsible for student clinical placements were recruited via organizational emails and invitations from NSH research team members. Informed consent was obtained verbally (interviews/focus groups) or electronically (survey) prior to any data collection. Maximum variation, non-probability volunteer sampling was used. Student participants were purposively selected for maximum variation by having them complete a short questionnaire using an online Microsoft Form, asking them to identify the faculty in which they were enrolled, program of study, year of study, and preference to participate in an interview or focus group.

To facilitate analysis, programs were categorized as early or late based on their curriculum structure. Early programs included students in year 1 of a 2-year program, year 1–2 of a 4-year program, and semesters 1–4 of an 8-semester program. Late programs included students in year 2 of a 2-year program, year 3–4 of a 4-year program, and semesters 5–8 of an 8-semester program. Participants were almost equally distributed between the early (52.1%) versus late (47.9%) program categories.

Data Collection and Analysis

Data were collected via an environmental scan, student survey, and interviews/focus group. The data collection tools were created by the research team to obtain rigorous objective and subjective data. All data were analyzed separately before mixing.

Environmental Scan

Environmental scans assist in the review of current services and programs to identify service gaps, professional education/training needs, and quality improvement initiatives to inform program and policy development (Charlton et al., 2019). In April-May 2021, we conducted an environmental scan using an electronic inventory form to assess the number and length of SBL disruptions enacted by the FoH/FoM because of the public health restrictions imposed during the first wave of the pandemic. Information collected included the program name, dates of SBL suspension and reintroduction, number of days between SBL suspensions and reintroductions, and number of students affected by the decisions to suspend SBL. The electronic inventory was sent to SBL coordinators (faculty and/or staff who arrange clinical placements) across FoH and FoM programs. Descriptive analysis of inventory data provided an overview of pandemic-related restrictions on student SBL.

Survey

The anonymous online survey was conducted to understand the perceived impact of pandemic-related curricular changes (e.g., suspension of SBL) on student learning, particularly during the first wave of the pandemic. The research team created survey questions based on recent literature about pandemic-related changes in higher education and our experiences as faculty and students. Questions were posed about: (1) participant experiences with online learning pre and post first wave of the pandemic, (2) changes and effectiveness of learning modalities, (3) SBL experiences, (4) confidence in performance of skills, (5) participation in extracurricular or volunteer pandemic response activities, (6) environment and resource availability for online learning, and (7) student support. Besides three demographic data questions (program of study, last year completed, age), the survey included 25 additional questions with a combination of question types, such as yes/no response items, open text boxes, 5-point Likert scales, and "select answers that apply." Completion of the survey was voluntary.

The survey was delivered using Opinio (<*https://www.objectplanet.com/opinio/*>), a secure web-based survey tool offered by Dalhousie University. Three weekly email reminders were sent as per the Dillman (2000) Strategy of Recruitment. The study aimed for the average web-based survey response rate of 34% or better (Shih & Fan, 2012). The survey data was analyzed with SPSS software v.27.

A detailed summary of Opinio raw survey data was downloaded into an Excel spreadsheet and was examined for incorrect, corrupted, incorrectly formatted, or duplicate data; none were noted. The detailed summary report was also examined for any missing data related to student choice not to answer a question prior to analysis. Analysis was conducted using descriptive statistics (to describe the characteristics of the data set in a meaningful way and identify emergent patterns in the data), sub-group analysis (to make comparisons between sub-groups of participants and investigate differences in how students responded), frequencies (to provide a visual representation of the distributions), and two-by-two Pearson Chi-Square Test of Independence (χ^2). The χ^2 statistic was performed to compare student cohorts (early versus late program categories) and pre-pandemic online learning with other variables identified in the survey (e.g., change of learning platforms) to test the association between the categorical variables to determine which categories may account for differences found (McHugh, 2013).

Interviews and Focus Group

The aim of the qualitative strand was to gain a deeper understanding of the impact of pandemic public health restrictions and the subsequent changes to teaching and students' learning, the existing policies and strategies used to overcome challenges caused by the pandemic, any barriers/risks that may have resulted, and suggestions of possible structures and processes to support decisions about the continuation of SBL during a pandemic. Semi-structured interview guides were developed by the research team to explore the perspectives and lived experiences of students, educators, and NSH managers/administrators. Verbatim interview and focus group transcripts were analyzed using thematic analysis in the coding software NVivo. Data from the interviews and the focus group were compared and reviewed through the systematic analysis of transcripts and indexing of data. Ongoing analysis was carried out through notetaking, reading, re-reading, and data reduction. To assure inter-coder reliability (Polit & Tatano Beck, 2012), three research team members (ME, NA, JL) independently reviewed two transcripts and discussed conflicts until consensus was reached. All transcripts were coded by these reviewers using a coding framework to organize findings into initial codes. A co-PI (ME) reviewed the data for emergent and cross cutting themes.

Results

Results of the environmental scan are offered first and separately from the qualitative and quantitative findings to demonstrate the disruptions per program to SBL in the FoH/FoM. Due to small sample sizes in the qualitative strand of the mixed methods study, saturation and thus identification of major themes was difficult to achieve. Therefore, the interview/focus group and survey open text question data are used as explanatory data sources to build on and explain the quantitative survey results, an approach supported by Creswell and Creswell (2017). Because the survey was voluntary and respondents could decide whether they wanted to answer a question, the percentages reported are based on the numbers of the outcomes of interests divided by the total number of respondents for each question.

Environmental Scan

SBL coordinators from 12 programs from the FoH (Appendix A) and one from the FoM (UGME) responded to the environmental scan inventory, representing 1159 students affected by SBL restrictions. On average, 89 students per program (with a range of 6–600 students) were impacted by the public health restrictions that changed face-to-face learning to online learning during the first wave of the pandemic. The number of days between amendments (e.g., canceling or pausing SBL) and reintroductions ranged from 63 to 395 days, with an approximate average of 152 days. The earliest date that SBL was amended was March 16, 2020; the latest date of initial amendment was July 1, 2020. The earliest date that students were reintroduced to SBL was May 20, 2020; however, the time frame for reintroduction was program dependent, extending to April 15, 2021, for two cohorts of learners (Appendix A).

Mixing of Data: Survey, Interviews, and Focus Group

Despite repeated and active recruitment methods, only 96 FoH and FoM students responded to the survey (3.2% response rate). A total of four interviews (*n* = 3 students; *n* = 1 educator) and one focus group (*n* = 3 educators) were conducted. No NSH key informants participated. Despite these small sample sizes, a wide range of health profession programs were represented. The number of respondents per program varied from 1 to 22; to maintain participant confidentiality, the frequency of participants per program is not reported. Nursing and medicine had the largest participation rates at 22.9% and 14.6%, respectively.

Online Learning Pre and Post First Wave Pandemic

During the first wave of the pandemic, 87.5% (n = 84/96) of respondents reported a change from face-to-face learning to online platforms. Among all respondents (N = 96), 76% (n = 73) had participated in online learning prior to the pandemic. Familiarity and use of online learning pre-pandemic were found to be significantly different (p < 0.001) between students in the early program category compared to those in the late program category. Students in the late program category (93.5%; n = 43/46) had more experience with online learning pre-pandemic compared to students in the early program category (60%; n = 30/50).

Changes and Effectiveness of Learning Modality

Two-thirds of participants (65.6%; n = 63/96) reported spending 0–3 hours per week on average in online SBL. When asked whether online SBL effectively replaced face-to-face SBL, only 13.5% (n = 13/96) agreed. Over one-third (36.5%; n = 35/96) of students disagreed that they could learn practical skills through online learning platforms, while 35.7% (n = 30/84) were unsure whether they could. There were no significant differences in positive versus negative impact on learning between students in the early and late program categories, although only 24.7% (n = 20/81) of students indicated that their learning was positively impacted by the change in modality, and 50.6% (n = 41/81) disagreed that it had. A nursing student shared that the change from face-to-face to online learning made them feel like they were learning on their own, "I feel like I'm basically teaching myself this entire program, … one of the most difficult courses I'm doing simply because of the structure, not the information or anything like that."

There were no significant differences between students who did or did not have a pre-pandemic online learning experience in online SBL [χ^2 (2, N = 84) = 0.71, p =.69] and their reported ability to learn skills online. Frequency analyses indicated that 40.9% (n = 27/66) of those with pre-pandemic online learning experiences and 44.4% (n = 8/18) of those without this experience disagreed that they could learn skills online.

Experiences with SBL

Synchronous simulation and lab-based online learning were rated as the most effective delivery methods for SBL (35.4%; n = 34/96) (Table 1). There were significant differences [χ^2 (14, N = 96) = 33.63, p = .002) between students with pre-pandemic online learning and those without in terms of identifying the most effective online learning delivery method. Among the 20 students who did not have previous pre-pandemic online learning experience, there were no preferred online delivery methods. However, among those with pre-pandemic online learning (n = 73/93), 46.6% (n = 34/73) chose synchronous simulation as the most effective.

Table 1: Most Effective Online Delivery Method for Skills-Based Learning

Delivery Method	Number (n)	Percentage (%)
Synchronous simulation/lab-based learning	34	35.4
Asynchronous lectures	13	13.5
Synchronous lectures	13	13.5
No response	10	10.4
Asynchronous learning materials/modules	9	9.4
Synchronous class discussion	7	7.3
Synchronous skill demonstration	7	7.3
Asynchronous skills demonstration	3	3.1

When asked whether their ability to learn skills had been affected during the pandemic, 42 out of the 81 respondents who answered this specific question (51.9%) reported that their learning was negatively affected, while 36 (44.4%) disagreed; 3 respondents (3.7%) neither agreed nor disagreed. One pharmacy student reported that recorded lectures were not as effective as the face-to-face setting:

> [Recorded lectures were] supposed to somewhat supplement the education that we didn't get when our hospital rotations got pushed. … We did a week of modules and stuff like that online … I would say I don't think it was as effective as in-person learning would have been.

A nursing student shared their negative online SBL experiences due to technological challenges, unrealistic time limits, and inadequate orientation to SBL devices:

> The timing is off a lot of the time … the technology being slow, you're trying to speak to somebody and there's a delay in their response. And when you're doing something where you only have seven minutes to get your point across, like they're timing you, [it's] quite significant … learning how to use all the devices and stuff, I thought really fell short.

Solely learning in online skills labs and a lack of patient exposure caused by the closure of practice setting sites (e.g., hospitals, LTC) during the first wave of the pandemic was perceived by students to negatively affect their skill development. One nursing student shared:

> There are certain things that you do in clinical … unless you do it on a real patient, it doesn't mean the same, doesn't make the same connection … it's not as good as if I had been able to do the thing in real life.

Another nursing student shared that interpersonal skill-building might suffer because of limited or no interactions with patients:

> I think therapeutic relationships … how to build that rapport with clients, I think that that's something that, you know, IV and catheter, you can learn about it wherever in the lab by practicing with your instructor. But I think people are scared to talk to the client.

Despite the identified limitations with online SBL, participants noted some positive experiences when interviewed. A pharmacy student explained:

> I felt like I was able to progress. And the recordings and stuff like having lectures online and being at home, I don't think it would be the case for everybody, but I really felt like it was nice to have recordings and stuff to lean on.

Confidence in Performance of Skills

Among all respondents (n = 78), 62.8% (n = 49) reported that their confidence in performing practical skills to a standard congruent to their level/stage of training had been affected by learning on an online platform. A total of 43 students out of 79 (54.4%) had concerns about their future ability to perform practical skills in their chosen profession. Students' confidence and concern with their future performance of program-specific skills showed no significant differences between early and late program categories, suggesting that regardless of the level of skill development (i.e., foundational skills in early programming versus advanced skills in later programming), student confidence was still impacted. There were no significant differences between students who did or did not have pre-pandemic online learning compared to their confidence to apply learned practical skills, but students with pre-pandemic online learning experience were more likely to acknowledge that their confidence was affected. A nursing student reflected on their lack of confidence in building collaborative and therapeutic relationships:

> Students are not comfortable around nurses or the interdisciplinary team. How to take ownership of the "how to," like pick up the call and answer a client's family call … they're scared of things like that. It was interesting to see because I think that just takes time. You need to be in a unit for long enough to be like, hey, I'm comfortable doing that.

Notwithstanding their lack of confidence, when asked if they believed they were at the skill level congruent with their level/stage of training, despite the transition to online learning, from a total of 75 responders, 54.7% (n = 41) agreed that they were, while 37.3 % (n = 28) disagreed, and 8.0% (n = 6) neither agreed nor disagreed. This suggests that even though a little over half of students lacked confidence in their perceived skills, almost the same number believed that they were at the level they should be at in their program for their actual skills. Faculty also acknowledged that students exhibited a loss of confidence in their perceived ability to perform skills as a result of the shift in SBL to online platforms. One educator described how students sometimes reacted to their clinical/fieldwork placements once resumed, regardless of whether they were new to the clinical environment or had been in clinical prior to the pandemic:

> They cried. … I had one group that was fresh, first placement, and a second group that was second placement. Somehow every placement, someone cries and then people get sick … people get stressed out. And one student told me that he wanted to quit nursing … it was very stressful. I spent a lot of time having long conversations to handle their emotions.

Faculty implemented strategies to lessen students' lack of confidence in their performance of skills. A nursing student described the supports faculty put in place to alleviate stress prior to students entering the clinical setting after restrictions were lifted:

> They started the semester a week early and that week was mainly focused on labs … I think it was two or three days. … We basically practiced almost every skill that we've done from the beginning. We got to go over those skills again because we had clinical starting in September … So, it was good to have that week where we went in.

Extracurricular/Volunteer Pandemic Response Activity

Some students (37.3%; n = 28/75) had participated in extracurricular and/or volunteer pandemic response activities. Survey responses indicate that these opportunities were predominantly sought out by students (57.2%; n = 16/29). Other ways that students learned about volunteer opportunities were through student associations, by students/peers sharing information, and/or directly from the institution offering the activity. Many students reported a lack of volunteer/extracurricular programming offered by their programs. When students did participate in extracurricular/volunteer pandemic response activities they utilized various platforms: online (14.3%; n = 4/28), in-person (64.3%; n = 18/28), or blended [online and in-person] (21.4%; n = 6/28). Although many students did not provide a response for the total number of weekly hours they participated in pandemic response activities, of the 73 who did, they reported working a range of hours (Table 2).

Table 2: Approximate Total Number of Hours Per Week for Pandemic Response Activities

Hours/week	Number (n)	Percentage (%)
<1	1	1.0
1–2	4	4.2
3–4	5	5.2
5–6	3	3.1
7–8	1	1.0
9–10	1	1.0
>10	7	7.3
N/A	1	1.0

When asked whether SBL in extracurricular or volunteer pandemic response activities had complemented their curricular learning, of those who responded (n = 28), 64.3% (n = 18) agreed that it had, whereas 21.4% (n = 6) disagreed, and 14.3% (n = 4) neither agreed nor disagreed. Practical skills relevant to their discipline were learned through extracurricular/volunteer pandemic response activities by 60.7% (n = 17/28) of respondents; however, 21.4% (n = 6/28) indicated that these experiences had not contributed to learning discipline-specific skills. Five students (17.9%) neither agreed nor disagreed. There were significant differences noted between students who had participated in extracurricular/volunteer activities with those who did not and their confidence (p = .013), suggesting that those who had participated in these activities were less likely to agree that their confidence in performing practical skills was negatively affected. Unfortunately, only a small number of participants (37.3%; n = 28/75) participated in these valuable experiences. When examining concerns for future performance, there was no significant difference between those with or without extracurricular/volunteer activities [χ^2 (4, N = 79) = 0.88, p = .9].

Environment and Resource Availability

Reliable computers and the internet were accessible to 98.7% (n = 75/76) of respondents; 95.9% (n = 71/74) of participants had access to videoconferencing software. Approximately two-thirds of the respondents had a quiet (70.7%; n = 53/75) and private (72.4%; n = 55/76) place to study. Despite many respondents having access and privacy, there were perceived problems with learning resources. One medical student shared that innovative and interactive ways to apply SBL were lacking:

> I found that with us being online, it was more of read this, read this, read this ... It was a lot of readings, but then there was no application. It was mainly recorded lectures as well, so you couldn't pause or stop to say, hey, can you explain this?

A pharmacy student suggested that to support students to learn skills virtually, interactive learning resources are needed at home, "I think it would be helpful to have the students have the materials in front of them, like say it's teaching the students how to use an inhaler or something … maybe send that stuff to the students."

Students also wanted more and clearer communication about clinical/fieldwork placements, inclusion in decision-making that affected them, better software for online skills training, and reliable resources to learn in a virtual world.

Discussion

This mixed methods study was conducted to better understand the impact of changes to FoH and FoM programs during the first wave of the pandemic. Findings are discussed under three broad areas: shifts in pedagogy, delivery of SBL, and challenges and solutions in skills performance. Strengths and limitations are presented. Implications in the form of academic, research, practice, and policy recommendations are offered.

Shifts in Pedagogy

There was variability in the responses to the pandemic from the programs analyzed, even though all were impacted and experienced cessation of activities and shifts from face-to-face learning to online platforms. The andragogical changes experienced at Dalhousie University followed a worldwide trend in promptly transitioning to virtual curricular delivery during the pandemic, with little consideration for the infrastructure, resource access, or digital competency required of students (Heng & Sol, 2021). While most participants indicated they had access to a computer and internet connection, quiet and private places to study were available to only half of the participants, findings that are in keeping with other studies (Heng & Sol, 2021; Ofori-Manteaw et al., 2022). Issues related to internet connectivity, access to technological devices, affordability of internet services, and student knowledge of how to use these resources and applications (i.e., digital competence) are cited as student concerns in the transition to online learning modalities (Heng & Sol, 2021; Ofori-Manteaw et al., 2022). Masha'al et al. (2020) reported that learning-related stressors experienced by nursing students were influenced by the type of electronic devices used to access online learning modalities, internet service type, and sociodemographic characteristics that impacted the availability of quiet, private places to study.

Delivery of SBL

Although most respondents identified synchronous simulation/labs as the most effective means to learn hands-on skills, one-third did not agree that it effectively replaced face-to-face learning, believing that their skill acquisition was negatively affected. This may be attributed in part to the technical difficulties of the online platform and/or missing opportunities to practice skills with real patients in clinical/fieldwork settings.

To replace hands-on SBL while in-person programming was restricted, FoH and FoM programs implemented creative ways to teach these skills through video-narrated demonstrations, small-group videoconferencing, virtual drop-in sessions, and online simulations, methods similar to those identified by Jeffries et al. (2022).

Students identified asynchronous and synchronous online lectures as the next most effective learning modalities, after synchronous online SBL, and reported that the use of these different delivery formats allowed time for them to engage in and reflect on the material while studying asynchronously. Similar to our findings, several authors have suggested that a mixture of asynchronous-synchronous formats maximizes the benefits of online learning (Ofori-Manteaw et al., 2022; Sen et al., 2021). These considerations are important to health professions education moving forward as some courses will undoubtedly remain in some type of blended synchronous-asynchronous format. Sen et al. (2021) report that simultaneous synchronous modalities allow for increased interaction between students and educators and promotes important socialization and feelings of connectivity, critical components to successful online learning (Bickle et al., 2019). In non-clinical UGME, Stojan et al. (2022) purport that the full potential of technology has yet to be fully realized and new developments must be informed by theory, evaluation outcomes, and provide details that support replication.

Challenges and Solutions in Skills Performance

Roughly half of the survey respondents believed that disruptions to learning and transition of SBL to virtual platforms affected their confidence to perform program-specific skills, leading to uncertainty about their future professional practice. Despite these beliefs, they perceived that their skill level was congruent with their stage of training. Both realities can be true at the same time because self-confidence is related to a person's judgment about *future* capabilities (Druckman & Bjork, 1994), whereas the question of whether they are at the skill level congruent with their level of training reflects current capabilities.

Educators also noted students' loss of confidence, resembling findings by Choi et al. (2020) who found that pandemic-related curricular changes impacted student readiness and confidence to transition to practice, especially since the introduction of virtual learning (Gaffney et al., 2021) and lack of hands-on training (Abbasi et al., 2020). Kaul et al. (2021) suggested that students may become more engaged in online learning, particularly with virtual reality (VR)-enhanced classroom settings and simulated clinical experiences as they are effective tools to consolidate learning (Saab et al., 2021) and increase confidence (Rushton et al., 2020). This suggests that computer-based learning to simulate clinical experiences may be valuable, giving students the opportunity to visualize content while at the same time interacting with it.

While volunteerism was not previously recognized as a valuable teaching tool (Chawlowska et al., 2021), perspectives may have shifted during the pandemic. Students were engaged as volunteer frontline healthcare workers in Ireland (Strawbridge et al., 2022), Italy (Villa et al., 2022), and the United Kingdom (Choi et al., 2020). Kaul et al. (2021) argue that student engagement with clinical or non-clinical volunteer/extracurricular duties may contribute to experiential learning. Choi et al. (2020) surmise that volunteering in pandemic response activities benefit students through mentorship and building empathy and patient-centeredness skills. Through these activities, students can gain new social, organizational, stress management skills, patient-provider communication, community links, interprofessional collaboration, and realistic perspectives of the healthcare system (Chalowska et al., 2021).

Our findings support extracurricular/volunteer pandemic response activities as beneficial and complementary to SBL. Students who engaged in these activities were less likely to feel that their confidence in practical skills was negatively affected. However, only one-quarter of surveyed students participated in such activities due to lack of awareness, confidence, motivation, and activities not meeting academic credit requirements (Chawlowska et al., 2021). Facilitating student participation in volunteer/extracurricular activities by quickly identifying opportunities, enhancing availability, and recognizing participation through formal credit might help mitigate students' low confidence in performing skills. It should also be noted that not all students may be able to participate in these extracurricular/volunteer experiences, and as such it is important that their inability does not place them at any disadvantage (e.g., applying to competitive positions or specialties).

Health professions students must master specific competencies to become safe practitioners to meet population healthcare needs. SBL is an essential teaching approach to ensure that this happens through a variety of ways, including volunteerism/extracurricular activities. Using the SBHHRP framework

(Tomblin Murphy et al., 2013), we focused on the impact the pandemic might have had on health professions education and the production of future HCPs available to the healthcare system to meet population needs (Lackie & Tomblin Murphy, 2020). Production considers students' educational characteristics—the knowledge, skills and abilities students attain before entering the workforce. How students are educated directly affects the competencies they attain and how they will contribute to future health services delivery (Lackie & Tomblin Murphy, 2020).

The results of this study show the importance of flexibility in response to interruptions in health professions education during a pandemic. A balance must be struck between ensuring programs continue to meet educational and regulatory standards while ensuring that the needs of society for safe, high-quality care are being met.

Strengths and Limitations

The interprofessional mix of researchers and students on the research team was helpful to develop data collection tools to understand the impact of pandemic-related curricular changes on health professions students' learning during the first wave of the pandemic. Another strength is that findings from the environmental scan provide timelines per program of when SBL was suspended and reintroduced, information that is critical to identify, monitor, and evaluate decision-making that positively or negatively impacted student learning outcomes.

Challenges were experienced in recruiting student and educator participants from each program. The low participation rates are likely due to a loss of interest in engaging in research because of multiple and persistent requests for participation, especially during the pandemic. This phenomenon is known as research (or participation) fatigue (Patel et al., 2020). There were low rates of return for surveys across all programs in both faculties, and we postulate that this may also be due to a combination of pandemic-related factors, such as changes to online learning, increased demands on time, and feelings of disengagement. The low survey sample size prevents the generalization of study findings to other academic units; however, qualitative data supports the quantitative findings; hence, there may be considerations from the mixed findings that will be applicable to other health professions schools and decision-makers moving forward. Another noted limitation was the large degree of variability among all aspects of the different programs surveyed, including size, direct (no prior university or college degree) versus graduate (previous university or college degree) program admission, length of training required, and timing of clinical and non-clinical rotations within each program.

Recommendations

Recommendations for consideration, garnered from study participants and current literature, are offered in hopes that the broader academic and healthcare communities may consider them in ways that support teaching and learning.

Academic

Students and educators advised that investments in human resources, infrastructure (space, equipment), and processes were required as they are essential for virtual SBL and in-person simulation-based education. INACSL et al. (2021) offer standards of best practice for simulation that align with the advice given by participants, including having personnel who are adept in information technology, mannikin operations and programming, and standardized patient education and coordination.

Investment in facilities and resources that support digital transformation, literacy, and competency of students and faculty were identified by study participants and supported by current literature (Heng & Sol, 2021). Research suggests that faculty need to build capacity to develop innovative teaching and assessment methods that align with digital instruction to increase student engagement (Heng & Sol, 2021; Stojan et al., 2022), findings that mirror feedback from participants in our study. Faculty development, provision of digital resources, technology support, and infrastructure to promote interactivity in the virtual world is crucial to the success of teaching and learning (Bastos et al., 2022).

To address student recommendations for at-home skills practice, academic programs should consider providing program-specific lab kits containing necessary supplies, which could be funded through student fees, to overcome resource accessibility issues during lockdowns and closures.

Students shared that they experienced stress about their ability to perform skills and the rapid shift to online SBL. Clearer and more timely communication with and between students and faculty regarding changes is warranted. Student representatives should be included in any decision-making that significantly impacts their learning.

Practice

Opportunity for students to practice program-specific skills beyond online and simulation environments is essential to develop higher order thinking skills (e.g., diagnosis, care management, and clinical judgment) (Australian Health Practitioner Regulation Agency [Ahpra] et al., 2021). Allowing students into practice settings during pandemics may mitigate potential negative downstream impacts of disruption to student SBL in clinical/fieldwork settings (e.g., student stress, unsafe practices). Ahpra et al. (2021) offered national principles for clinical education during the pandemic that may be beneficial for Canadian health professions schools, practice settings, and regulatory bodies to consider. These recommendations emphasize the need to balance short and long-term risks, ensure student safety, prioritize senior students for placements, adopt flexible learning approaches, improve communication and collaboration with stakeholders, consider optimal utilization of student skills, monitor and manage risks, and acknowledge learning gained through paid employment.

Research

Findings highlighted the stressors that students faced during suspensions to in-person learning which impacted their confidence; however, educators' stress was not considered. Rabe et al. (2020) found that faculty experienced increased mental, emotional, and physical health issues such as stress and confusion during the pandemic. Investigations about educator experiences, with the goal of identifying support strategies, are warranted.

Students felt a loss of confidence in their ability to perform skills and worried about their future performance; however, since we did not assess student skills, we do not know whether their perceptions were reality. Further investigation is needed to explore how students and faculty manage expectations of performance during highly stressful events and whether student performance declined because of the curricular changes.

Because there were such large degrees of variation between programs, future research that explores program-specific impacts caused by pandemic-related curriculum changes may provide detailed and distinct program planning information. There is a need for high-quality, cross-sectional, and longitudinal studies to provide robust examination of the effects of the pandemic on student learning.

Policy

Despite many years of predicting a global pandemic, the world was not ready to face such an international crisis (Ali Jadoo, 2020). Alert systems, crisis management practices, and community, national, and global policies and plans were either non-existent, ineffective, or flawed. Findings from our study, while admittedly at a local level (e.g., Nova Scotia), identifies the unpreparedness experienced by academic institutions and service partners to respond to the impact posed to student learning by public health restrictions. As such, we recommend the creation of evidence-informed intersectoral policies and concrete mechanisms to guide future pandemic response activities associated with continuation of student SBL. Policies, as well as their coordinated usage, are required to guide extracurricular/volunteer pandemic response activities, as well as the continuation of SBL with service partners. Regulatory bodies, who determine entry-level competencies for their respective professions, must be consulted to help determine which activities could be considered toward academic credit.

Conclusion

Notwithstanding the limitations of this study, findings have provided some insights into pandemic-related SBL for the academic, practice, research, and policy communities in Nova Scotia. Findings highlighted the challenges faced by academic institutions when responding to public health restrictions and the resultant impacts on health professional student SBL. Programs implemented different strategies to address the restrictions, such as staggering disruptions to clinical placements by cohort, shifting to online learning platforms, and suspending face-to-face SBL. However, despite these various strategies, students' confidence in their future skills performance declined. Synchronous simulation emerged as the most effective online learning method for SBL, though some students faced challenges with finding a suitable study environment. It is speculated that allowing students into practice settings during a pandemic may mitigate potential negative effects of the disruption of SBL, as online learning alone may not be sufficient. Engagement in extracurricular healthcare activities helped some students to alleviate concerns with their future practice of skills. Volunteer opportunities for students to help the community as frontline workers may also be encouraged, with the caveat that students who are unable to volunteer would not be penalized. It is recommended that evidence-based policies be created to ensure that students, educators, and health education institutions are prepared to handle future crises that disrupt health professions education. Recognizing that the study was conducted at one university, recommendations offered may not be relevant or appropriate across different contexts. However, analyzing the measures taken to resolve issues related to students' SBL during the pandemic and their results may assist those who plan for future waves of this pandemic and others.

Bibliography

Abbasi, M. S., Ahmed, N., Sajjad, B., Alshahrani, A., Saeed, S., Sarfaraz, S., Alhamdan, R. S., Vohra, F., & Abduljabbar, T. (2020). E-learning perception and satisfaction among health sciences students amid the COVID-19 pandemic. *Work, 67*(3), 549–556. <https://doi.org/10.3233/WOR-203308>

Ali Jadoo, S. A. (2020, May 19). Was the world ready to face a crisis like COVID-19? *Jidhealth, 3*(1), 123–4. <https://www.jidhealth.com/index.php/jidhealth/article/view/45>

Alsoufi, A., Alsuyihili, A., Msherghi, A., Elhadi, A., Atiyah, H., Ashini, A., Ashwieb, A., Ghula, M., Ben Hasan, H., Abudabuos, S., Alameen, H., Abokhdhir, T., Anaiba, M., Nagib, T., Shuwayyah, A., Benothman, R., Arrefae, G., Alkhwayildi, A., Alhadi, A., ... Elhadi, M. (2020). Impact of the COVID-19 pandemic on medical education: Medical students' knowledge, attitudes, and practices regarding electronic learning. *PLOS ONE, 15*(11), e0242905. <https://doi.org/10.1371/journal.pone.0242905>

Australian Health Practitioner Regulation Agency (Ahpra) & National Boards. (2021, Aug 27). *National principles for clinical education during COVID-19.* <https://www.ahpra.gov.au/Resources/COVID-19/National-principles-for-clinical-education-during-COVID-19.aspx>

Bastos, R. A., Carvalho, D. R. dos S., Brandão, C. F. S., Bergamasco, E. C., Sandars, J., & Cecilio-Fernandes, D. (2022). Solutions, enablers and barriers to online learning in clinical medical education during the first year of the COVID-19 pandemic: A rapid review. *Medical Teacher, 44*(2), 187–195. <https://doi.org/10.1080/0142159X.2021.1973979>

Bickle, M. C., Rucker, R. D., & Burnsed, K. A. (2019). Online learning: Examination of attributes that promote student satisfaction. *Online Journal of Distance Learning Administration, XXII* (1), 1–7.

Boshra, B. (2020, April 16). *Quebec order allows health-care students near graduation, recent retirees to work during COVID-19 pandemic.* CTV News. <https://montreal.ctvnews.ca/quebec-order-allows-health-care-students-near-graduation-recent-retirees-to-work-during-covid-19-pandemic-1.4898614>

British Columbia College of Nursing Professionals. (2020). *Employed student nurses.* <https://www.bccnm.ca/RN/applications_registration/how_to_apply/ESR_RN/Pages/Default.aspx>

Canadian Association of Schools of Nursing. (2020). *Nursing education during the COVID-19 pandemic.* <https://www.casn.ca/wp-content/uploads/2020/03/COVID-19-POSITION-STATEMENT.pdf>

Charlton, P., Doucet, S., Azar, R., Nagel, D. A., Boulos, L., Luke, A., Mears, K., Kelly, K. J., & Montelpare, W. J. (2019). The use of the environmental scan in health services delivery research: A scoping review protocol. *BMJ Open, 9*(9), e029805. <https://doi.org/10.1136/bmjopen-2019-029805>

Chawlowska, E., Staszewski, R., Lipiak, A., Giernas, B., Karasiewicz, M., Bazan, MD., Nowosadko, M., Cofta, M., & Wysocki, J. (2021). Student volunteering as a solution for undergraduate health professions education: Lessons from the COVID-19 pandemic. *Frontiers in Public Health, 8*(633888), 1–11. <https://doi.org/10.3389/fpubh.2020.633888>

Chief Medical Officer of Health. (2021, May 8). *Restated order #2 of the Chief Medical Officer of Health under Section 32 of the Health Protection Act 2004 (c.4, s.1).* Nova Scotia Legislature. <http://mcmillan.ca/wp-content/uploads/2020/09/health-protection-act-order-by-the-medical-officer-of-health.pd_.pdf.>

Choi, B., Jegatheeswaran, L., Minocha, A., Alhilani, M., Nakhoul, M., & Mutengesa, E. (2020). The impact of the COVID-19 pandemic on final year medical students in the United Kingdom: A national survey. *BMC Medical Education, 20*(206), 1–11. <https://doi.org/10.1186/s12909-020-02117-1>

College of Nurses of Ontario. (2020). *COVID-19 Information.* <https://www.cno.org/en/covid-19/novel-coronavirus/>

Cooke A. (2022). Dalhousie nursing students told to work in long-term care rather than do clinical practicum. Global News. <https://globalnews.ca/news/8542768/dalhousie-nursing-long-term-care-practicum/>

Creswell, J. W., & Creswell, J. D. (2017). *Research design: Qualitative, quantitative, and mixed methods approaches.* Sage publications.

Creswell, J. W., & Plano Clark, V. L. (2018). *Designing and conducting mixed methods research.* (3rd ed.). Sage Publications.

Dalhousie University Faculty of Health (2023). *Programs.* <https://www.dal.ca/faculty/health/programs.html>

Dedeilia, A., Sotiropoulos, M. G., Hanrahan, J. G., Janga, D., Dedeilias, P., & Sideris, M. (2020). Medical and surgical education challenges and innovations in the COVID-19 era: A systematic review. *In Vivo, 34*(3 suppl), 1603–1611. <https://doi.org/10.21873/invivo.11950>

Dillman, D. A. (2000). *Mail and internet surveys: The tailored design.* John Wiley & Sons, Inc.

Druckman, D. & Bjork, R. A. (1994). Self-confidence and performance. In D. Druckman & R. A. Bjork (Eds.), *Learning, remembering, believing: Enhancing human performance* (pp. 173–206). National Academy Press.

Foroozan, T. (2020). Nearly graduated nursing students fast-tracked into service after COVID-19 crisis cut practicums short. CBC News. <https://www.cbc.ca/news/canada/calgary/nurses-covid-pandemic-calgary-fast-track-rn-mru-1.5532816>

Gaffney, M. K., Chargualaf, K. A., & Ghosh, S. (2021). COVID-19 disruption of nursing education and the effects on students' academic and professional confidence. *Nurse Educator 46*(2), 76–81. <https://doi.org/10.1097/NNE.0000000000000986>

Gorman, M. (2020). *N. S. regulators for doctors, nurses clear path for reinforcements amid COVID-19.* CBC News. <https://www.cbc.ca/news/canada/nova-scotia/covid-19-health-care-doctors-nurses-medicine-hospitals-1.5500767>

Heng, K. & Sol, K. (2021). Online learning during COVID-19: Key challenges and suggestions to enhance effectiveness. *Cambodian Journal of Educational Research, 1*(1), 3–16. <http://www.cefcambodia.com/>

INACSL Standards Committee, Charnetski, M., & Jarvill, M. (2021, September). Healthcare Simulation Standards of Best Practice TM Operations. *Clinical Simulation in Nursing, 58*, 33–39. <https://doi.org/10. 1016/j.ecns.2021.08.012>

Jeffries, P. R., Bushardt, R. L., DuBose-Morris, R., Hood, C., Kardong-Edgren, S., Pintz, C., Posey, L., & Sikka, N. (2022). The role of technology in health professions education during the COVID-19 pandemic. *Academic Medicine, 97*(3S), S104-S109. <https://doi.org/10.1097/ACM.0000000000004523>

Kaul, V., de Moraes, A. G., Khateeb, D., Greenstein, Y., Winter, G., Chae, J. M., Stewart, N. H., Qadir, N., & Dangayach, N. S. (2021). Medical education during the COVID-19 pandemic. *Chest, 159*(5), 1949–1960. <https://doi.org/10.1016/j.chest.2020.12.026>

Lackie, K., & Tomblin Murphy, G. (2020). The impact of interprofessional collaboration on productivity: Important considerations in health human resources planning. *Journal of Interprofessional Education & Practice, 21*, 1–8. <https://doi:10.1016/j.xjep.2020.100375>

Masha'al D., Rababa, M., & Shahrour, G. (2020). Distance learning–related stress among undergraduate nursing students during the COVID-19 pandemic. *Journal of Nursing Education, 59*(12), 666–674. <https://doi.org/10.3928/01484834-20201118-03>

McFadden, S., Guille, S., Daly-Lynn, J., O'Neill, B., Marley, J., Hanratty, C., Shepard, P., Ramsey, L., Breen, C., Duffy, O., Jones, A., Kerr, D., & Hughes, C. (2022). Academic, clinical, and personal experiences of undergraduate healthcare students during the COVID-19 pandemic: A prospective cohort study. *PLOS One, 17*(7), e0271873 <https://doi.org/10.1371/journal.pone.0271873>

McHugh, M. L. (2013). The Chi-square test of independence. *Biochem Med, 23*(2), 143–149. <https://doi.org/10.11613%2FBM.2013.018>

Merritt, B. (2020, June 20a). Message from the Dean. *Dal Health messages regarding COVID-19.* <*https://www.dal.ca/faculty/health/newsevents/news/2020/03/23/dal_health_dean_covid19.html*>

Merritt, B. (2020, August 11b). COVID-19 update. Dal Health messages regarding COVID-19. <*https://www.dal.ca/faculty/health/news-events/news/2020/03/23/dal_health_dean_covid19.html*>

Nova Scotia Health Authority. (2023). *About Nova Scotia Health.* <https://www.nshealth.ca/about-nova-scotia-health>

Ofori-Manteaw, B. B., Dzidzornu, E., & Akudjedu, T. N. (2022). Impact of the COVID-19 pandemic on clinical radiography education: Perspective of students and educators from a low resource setting. *Journal of Medical Imaging & Radiation Sciences, 53*(1), 51–57. <https://doi.org/10.1016/j.jmir.2021.11.002>

Ontario Physiotherapy Association. (2022). Where we stand. <https://opa.on.ca/advocacy-positions/where-we-stand/>

Patel, S. S., Webster, R. K., Greenberg, N., Weston, D., & Brooks, S. K. (2020). Research fatigue in COVID-19 pandemic and post-disaster research: Causes, consequences and recommendations. *Disaster Prevention and Management: An International Journal, 29*(4), 445–455. <https://doi.org/10.1108/DPM-05-2020-0164>

Polit, D. F. & Tatano Beck, C. (2012). *Nursing research. Generating and assessing evidence for nursing practice* (9th ed.). Wolters Kluwer Health/Lippincott Williams & Wilkins.

Rabe, A., Sy, M., Cheung, W. Y. W., & Lucero-Prisno, D. E. (2020). COVID-19 and health professions education: A 360°view of the impact of a global health emergency [version 1]. *MedEdPublish.* <https://mededpublish.org/articles/9-148>

Rushton, M. A., Drumm, I. A., Campion, S. P., & O'Hare, J. J. (2020). The use of immersive and virtual reality technologies to enable nursing students to experience scenario-based, basic life support training—exploring the impact on confidence and skills. *CIN: Computers, Informatics, Nursing, 38*(6), 281–293, <https://doi.org/10.1097/CIN.0000000000000608>

Saab, M. M., Hegarty, J., Murphy, D., & Landers, M. (2021). Incorporating virtual reality in nursing education: A qualitative study of nursing students' perspectives. *Nurse Education Today, 105*(105045), 1–7. <https://doi.org/10.1016/j.nedt.2021.105045>

Sen, S. K., Edwards Collins, M. E., & Ingram, C. D. (2021). Innovative strategies for occupational therapy education delivery during coronavirus disease 2019 and beyond: A perspective. *Indian Journal of Occupational Therapy (Wolters Kluwer India Pvt Ltd), 53*(4), 161–164. <https://doi.org/10.4103/ijoth.ijoth_63_21>

Shih, T.-H., & Fan, X. (2012). Comparing response rates from web and mail surveys: A meta-analysis. *Field Methods, 20*(3), 249–271. <https://doi.org/10.1177/1525822X08317085>

Smith, E. (2020, May 8). Dal medical student volunteers to help at epicentre of N. S. COVID-19 outbreak. *CBC News*. <https://www.cbc.ca/news/canada/nova-scotia/northwood-halifax-medical-student-volunteer-long-term-care-1.5562222>

Stojan, J., Haas, M., Thammasitboon, S., Lander, L., Evans, S., Pawlik, C., Pawilkowska, T., Lew, M., Khamees, D., Peterson, W., Hider, A., Grafton-Clarke, C., Uraiby, H., Gordon, M., & Daniel, M. (2022). Online learning developments in undergraduate medical education in response to the COVID-19 pandemic: A BEME systematic review: BEME Guide No. 69. *Medical Teacher, 44*(2), 109–129. <https://doi.org/10.1080/01421 59X.2021.1992373>

Stout, R. C., Roberts, S., Maxwell-Scott, H., & Gothard, P. (2021). Necessity is the mother of invention: How the COVID-19 pandemic could change medical student placements for the better. *Postgraduate Medical Journal, 97*(1149), 417–422. <https://doi.org/10.1136/postgradmedj-2021-139728>

Strawbridge, J., Hayden, J. C., Robson, T., Flood, M., Cullinan, S., Lynch, M., Morgan, A. T., O'Brien, F., Reynolds, R., Kerrigan, S. W., Cavalleri, G., Kirby, B. P., Tighe, O., Maher, A., & Barlow, J. W. (2022). Educating pharmacy students through a pandemic: Reflecting on our COVID-19 experience. *Administrative Pharmacy, 18*(7), 3204–3209. <https://doi.org/10.1016/j.sapharm.2021.08.007>

Tomblin Murphy, G. (2007). *A framework for collaborative Pan-Canadian health human resources planning. Appendix: Example of a conceptual model for HHR planning. Government of Canada*. <http://www.hc-sc.gc.ca/hcs-sss/pubs/hhrhs/2007-frame-cadre/app-ann-eng.php>

Tomblin Murphy, G., MacKenzie, A., Alder, R., Langley, J., Hickey, M. & Cook, A. (2013). Pilot-testing an applied competency-based approach to health human resources planning. *Health Policy and Planning, 28* (7), 739–749.

Villa, G., Galli, E., Allieri, S., Baldrighi, R., Brunetti, A., Gianetta, N., & Manara, D. F. (2022). Frontline involvement in population COVID-19 vaccinations: Lived experiences of nursing students. *Healthcare 2022, 10*(1985), 1–11. <https://doi.org/10.3390/healthcare10101985>

Williams, G. A., Maier, C. B., Scarpetti, G., Giulio de Belvis, A., Fattore, G., Morsella, A., Pastorino, G., Poscia, A., Ricciardi, W., & Silenzi, A. (2020). What strategies are countries using to expand health workforce surge capacity during the COVID-19 pandemic? *Eurohealth 26(2)*, 51–57.

Appendix A

Program Amendments to SBL During COVID-19

Program	Date made to amend SBL	Date made to reintroduce SBL	Days between amendment and reintroduction to SBL	Number of students affected
Audiology	March 16, 2020	September 14, 2020	182	30
Clinical Vision Science	March 19, 2020	June 8, 2020	81	6
Diagnostic Medical Ultrasound (2017 intake)	March 16, 2020	June 8, 2020	84	6
Diagnostic Medical Ultrasound (2018 intake)	March 16, 2020	September 8, 2020	176	7
Diagnostic Medical Ultrasound (2019 intake)	March 16, 2020	September 8, 2020	176	7
Diagnostic Medical Ultrasound (2020 intake)	July 1, 2020	September 8, 2020	69	7
Medical Doctor (undergraduate medicine)	March 18, 2020	June 8, 2020	82	84
MRI 2019 intake (also Nuclear Medicine 2016 intake)	March 16, 2020	June 8, 2020	84	5
Nuclear Medicine (2017 intake)	March 16, 2020	September 8, 2020	176	7

Program	Date made to amend SBL	Date made to reintroduce SBL	Days between amendment and reintroduction to SBL	Number of students affected
Nuclear Medicine (2018 intake)	March 16, 2020	September 8, 2020	176	7
Nuclear Medicine (2019 intake)	March 16, 2020	April 15, 2021	395	7
Nuclear Medicine (2020 intake)	July 1, 2020	April 15, 2021	288	7
Nursing	April 15, 2020	September 1, 2020	139	384
Occupational Therapy	March 16, 2020	June 23, 2020	99	66–132
Pharmacy	March 18, 2020	January 4, 2021	292	360
Radiological Technology (2016 intake)	March 16, 2020	N/A		13
Radiological Technology (2017 intake)	March 16, 2020	September 8, 2020	176	12
Radiological Technology (2018 intake)	March 16, 2020	September 8, 2020	176	11
Radiological Technology (2019 intake)	March 16, 2020	September 8, 2020	176	13
Radiological Technology (2020 intake)	July 1, 2020	September 8, 2020	69	13
Respiratory Therapy (2017 intake)	March 16, 2020	June 8, 2020	84	10

(Continued)

(*Continued*)

Program	Date made to amend SBL	Date made to reintroduce SBL	Days between amendment and reintroduction to SBL	Number of students affected
Respiratory Therapy (2018 intake)	March 16, 2020	September 8, 2020	176	13
Respiratory Therapy (2019 intake)	March 16, 2020	September 8, 2020	176	12
Respiratory Therapy (2020 intake)	July 1, 2020	September 8, 2020	69	12
Social Work (total number of students included in above)	March 18, 2020	May 20, 2020	63	
Social Work (with Occupational Therapy and Therapeutic Recreation in an IP clinic)	March 20, 2020	August 10, 2020	145	600
Speech Language Pathology	March 16, 2020	July 27, 2020	133	52
TOTAL				1159

CONTRIBUTORS

JEFF KARABANOW is Professor and Associate Director at the School of Social Work at Dalhousie University. He has worked with people experiencing homelessness in Toronto, Montreal, Halifax, and Guatemala. He is also a recent awardee of the Senate of Canada 150 Medal.

JEAN HUGHES is Professor at the School of Nursing at Dalhousie University. Her research and publications concentrate on populations who are marginalized with a focus on mental health, many including homeless populations. She has scientific appointments with IWK Children's Hospital and Nova Scotia Health.

HAORUI WU is Canada Research Chair (Tier II) in Resilience and Associate Professor in the School of Social Work at Dalhousie University. His community-based interdisciplinary efforts examine human-animal-environment interplay through the lens of environmental, social, and health justice in disaster settings.

CATHERINE LEVITEN-REID is Associate Professor in the MBA in Community Economic Development program at Cape Breton University. Catherine does research on affordable housing, homelessness, and the social economy, primarily in partnership with community-based organizations. She also leads a Community University Housing Research Lab.

GRACE SKAHAN is completing her Ph.D. in the Department of Integrated Studies in Education at McGill University. Grace holds a Master of Arts in Education from McGill, and her research interests include gender-based violence prevention, masculinities, and participatory and arts-based education and research.

S. M. HANI SADATI is Senior Researcher at the Center for Community-Based Research, located at the University of Waterloo, Canada. He completed his Ph.D. in Educational Studies at McGill University, where his research focused on game-based learning. Hani specializes in community-based research.

SHANNON ROY is a Ph.D. candidate at McGill University's Department of Integrated Studies in Education, focusing on teacher identity, feminist theory, and arts-based research. Her exploration centers on the transformative potential of photography and cellphilming as tools to unearth educators' and students' narratives, to enhance educational practices.

CLAUDIA MITCHELL is Distinguished James McGill Professor at McGill University, where she is the Director of the Institute for Human Development and Well-being and the Founder and Director of the Participatory Cultures Lab. Her work addresses visual methodologies, girlhood studies, gender, and social justice.

DAWN ZINGA is Professor of Child and Youth Studies at Brock University who researches mental health and social interactions among youth within schools, community contexts, and activities such as dance. Her research has been supported by the Social Sciences and Humanities Research Council of Canada.

DANIELLE S. MOLNAR is Tier II Canada Research Chair in Adjustment and Well-Being in Children and Youth and an Associate Professor in the Department of Child and Youth Studies at Brock University. Dr. Molnar's multidisciplinary program of research aims to understand perfectionism among youth.

MELISSA BLACKBURN is a Ph.D. candidate in the Department of Child and Youth Studies at Brock University. Melissa's multi-method program of research focuses on how perfectionism among young people contributes to well-being outcomes, including psychopathology, physical health, psychosocial functioning, and academic experiences.

NATALIE TACURI is a Ph.D. candidate in the Department of Integrated Studies in Education & Institute for Gender, Sexuality and Feminist Studies at McGill University. Natalie's research interests include dance education, girlhood studies, sexualization, student-athletes, and feminist theories and methodologies.

OLIVIA LESLIE HOLDEN, MA, is a doctoral student in the School/Applied Child Psychology program at McGill University. Broadly, her research focuses on child sexual abuse disclosure and sibling relationships.

ANNIE YUN AN SHIAU, MA, is a doctoral student in the School/Applied Child Psychology program at McGill University. She is broadly interested in forensic interviewing protocols and cross-cultural examination of sexual abuse disclosures.

SHAYLA CHILLIAK is a Ph.D. student in School and Applied Child Psychology at McGill University. Her research interests include best practices for interviewing asylum-seeking youth, improving child maltreatment identification and response, social media and youth mental health, and interventions supporting sexually and gender diverse youth.

VICTORIA TALWAR is Professor and Canada Research Chair (Tier 1) in Forensic Developmental Psychology in the Department of Educational & Counseling Psychology at McGill University. Her research examines issues related to child witness disclosures and testimony.

SHANNA DEWIT WILLIAMS is Assistant Professor in the Department of Educational and Counseling Psychology at McGill University. She has worked with maltreated populations while conducting forensic interviews for various law enforcement agencies in the United States and Canada.

KELLY LACKIE, Ph.D., RN, CCSNE, is Associate Professor and the Associate Director of Simulation-based Education and Interprofessional Education in the School of Nursing at Dalhousie University. Her research is situated in interprofessional education, collaborative practice, and psychological safety, examined through equity, diversity, inclusion, and accessibility lens.

NEDA ALIZADEH, B.Sc. OT, M.Sc. OT, Ph.D. in Health, specializes in developing and evaluating patient-oriented health interventions for neurological conditions. Additionally, her research interests focus on substance use disorders, mental health, and health equity. She is an expert in mixed methods research and scoping reviews.

MARK EMBRETT is Lead Implementation Scientist at Nova Scotia Health, spearheading the analysis and implementation of strategies across the health system, including proof-of-concept projects for provincial health innovations. Mark also leads rapid evidence synthesis to inform innovative health policies and strategies.

SIMON FIELD is Professor and Head of the Department of Emergency Medicine at Dalhousie University. He works as an Emergency Physician in Halifax, and has interests in distributed education, assessment of learners, and critical thinking.

JENNIFER LANE, Ph.D., RN, is Assistant Professor at Dalhousie University's School of Nursing. Dr. Lane is a health equity researcher who utilizes Intersectionality Theory to explore the impacts of contextual power relations on access to and the delivery of health and social services.

MARION BROWN is a social worker, educator, and Associate Dean Academic in the Faculty of Health at Dalhousie University. She provides strategic leadership in program and curriculum development, implementation, evaluation, and continuous improvement for academic and scholarly innovation, and was awarded the 2024 Dalhousie Award of Excellence for Teaching.

DIANE MACKENZIE, Ph.D., OT Reg (NS), is Associate Professor in the School of Occupational Therapy, the Interprofessional Health Education Coordinator for the Faculty of Health at Dalhousie University, and an Affiliated Scientist with Nova Scotia Health. Her research interests include health profession education, simulation, and neurorehabilitation.

BRIGHT HUO is a general surgery resident at McMaster University. His clinical interests are in foregut surgery, specifically in the surgical management of gastroesophageal reflux disease. His research interests relate to the development of clinical practice guidelines and the clinical integration of large language models.

KATHLEEN MACMILLAN, B.Sc. Pharm, MD, is a radiology resident at Dalhousie University in Halifax, Nova Scotia. Kathleen is involved in a broad range of leadership and research activities. She currently serves on the boards of both Maritime Resident Doctors and the Canadian Association of Radiologists.

RUTH MARTIN-MISENER, NP, Ph.D., FAAN, FCAN, is Director and Professor at Dalhousie University School of Nursing and Co-Director of the Canadian Center for Advanced Practice Nursing at McMaster University. Her research focus is team-based models of healthcare, nurse practitioners, and other specialized nursing roles.